Praise for Jones' C

"*Confessions of a Trauma Junkie* is a book written from the heart. It reads like a collection of short stories, but these stories are not fictional. They come from real-life experiences. Some are funny; some are sad; some are hopeful, but all shine a light on a caring heart of a paramedic nurse who shows the deepest respect for human life in all its manifestations."

—Jeffrey T. Mitchell, Ph.D.
Clinical Professor of Emergency Health Services, University of Maryland, Baltimore County, President Emeritus, International Critical Incident Stress Foundation

"A must read for those who choose to subject themselves to life at its best and at its worst. Sherry offers insight in the Emergency Response business that most people cannot imagine. This book details life through the eyes of a caring individual who is a devoted CISM practitioner and true professional, who continually accepts the crisis presented, employs best practices, focuses on the mission, and makes the trauma, pain and suffering a little easier to manage."

—Maj Gen Richard L. Bowling,
former Commanding General, USAF Auxiliary (CAP)

"We are not alone. Sherry Jones shares experiences and unique personal insights of first responders. Told with poetry, sensitivity and a touch of humor at times, all are real, providing views into realities EMTs, Nurses, and other first responders encounter. Emotions shared bind this fraternity/sorority together in understanding, service and goals. Recommended reading for anyone working with trauma, crises, critical incidents in any profession. It's heartening to know we share such common experiences and support from our peers."

—George W. Doherty, MS, LPC, President
Rocky Mountain Region Disaster Mental Health Institute

"In this book, Sherry has captured the essence of working with people who have witnessed trauma. It made me cry, it made me laugh, it helped me to understand differently the work of our Emergency Services Personnel. I consider this a 'MUST READ' for all of us who wish to be helpful to those who work in these professions."
— Dennis Potter, LMSW, CAAC, FAAETS, ICISF Instructor

"*Confessions of a Trauma Junkie* is an honest, powerful and moving account of the emotional realities of helping others. Sherry Jones gives us a privileged look into the healing professions she knows firsthand. Her deep experience is a source of knowledge and inspiration for all who wish to serve. The importance of peer support is beautifully illustrated. This book will deepen the reader's respect for those who serve."
—Victor Welzant, PsyD
Director of Education and Training
The International Critical Incident Stress Foundation, Inc

"Never before has anyone depicted in such vivid detail the real life experiences of a street medic. EMS is a profession that at times can be extremely rewarding and other times painfully tragic. Thank you for telling our story through your eyes!"
—Diane F. Fojt, CEO
Corporate Crisis Management, Inc.
Former Flight Paramedic

"This true life documentation is an interesting look into the quality and care presented in the most traumatic incidents. All told, this book will bring a greater understanding of just how much these very special people are capable of, how caring they are, and why some burn out so soon. I definitely recommend this book on many levels. Who has not had some connection to this field at some point in their lives? This is how it is, written faithfully and dealing more with outcomes and feelings than with a gory tale. The book is very well written with a nice balance to hold the layperson's attention."
—Betty Gelean, *Nightreader*

"This is an extremely well written book. The author uses the English language in such an elegant manner the reader is sitting right there in the story without being so inundated with words that the story loses its meaning. The stories flow very nicely with just enough interjection from the author, to give background or explain terms to allow the reader to understand completely what is taking place."

—Melissa Koltes, *Rebecca's Reads*

"Through the venue of real and personable human experience stories, Sherry's *More Confessions* is a powerfully written sequel that provides key insights into the need for those who work in emergency and disaster response, as well as their families, to actively and purposely recognize and consistently address their physical, mental, and spiritual well-being. All who read this book will be touched deeply in some way."

—Harvey J. Burnett, Jr., PhD, LP,
President, Michigan Crisis Response Association
Sergeant, Buchanan Police Department
Assistant Prof. of Psychology, Behavioral Sciences Dept., Andrews University

"I found each essay to be incredibly compelling. Several also reminded me of similar situations that would occur at the hospitals that I worked at, especially the humorous ones. I was also reminded that in addition to dealing with the job stresses and long hours, each person also has to deal with their own personal issues. I highly recommend *Confessions of a Trauma Junkie* by Sherry Jones to nursing and EMT students. I think it should be required reading for them. I also recommend this book to people who are already working in the field. They will enjoy the stories and I believe that it will be reassuring to them to know that they are not alone in both their feelings and their experiences on the job."

—Paige Lovitt, *Reader Views*

"Sherry's first book *Confessions of a Trauma Junkie* opened my eyes to the realities of being an emergency services worker, especially as an EMT and a nurse paramedic. But Sherry has had a lifetime of experiences, and one book just wasn't enough to say everything, so now, *More Confessions of a Trauma Junkie* fulfills that need. This 'sequel' offers humor to anyone needing a laugh, insight into emergency services for anyone considering such a career, and I think for Sherry's colleagues, a comic and truthful look at the work they do every day to save lives. *But More Confessions of a Trauma Junkie* is more than a compilation of funny stories. It gets at the very heart of what it is to be an EMT, a paramedic, a nurse, or a doctor. It is a heroic, exhausting, and emotionally traumatic calling. Other people's trauma can become the emergency worker's trauma, even though the workers try very hard not to let these situations affect them. As Sherry points out, 'Rule #1: People Die. Rule #2: Medics cannot change rule #1. (But boy, do we try!')."

— Tyler R. Tichelaar, Ph.D.,
author of the award-winning *Narrow Lives*

"Life as a nurse or a paramedic is no easy task. They need to know their procedures and medical knowledge like the back of their hand. They need to be prepared mentally, physically and emotionally to deal with everything that comes through their doors on a daily (or hourly?) basis. Sherry Jones has been both, and in her book, *Confessions of a Trauma Junkie*, there are several essays and short stories that dive into her world: the tragic, the hopeful and the humorous. This book shows us a world that some of us know we could not be a part of. And maybe, will show you that yes, these people are people too, and they may understand how you are feeling."

—Margaret Orford, *Allbooks Reviews*

More Confessions of a Trauma Junkie

My Life as a Nurse Paramedic -

Folie à Deux

2nd Edition

Sherry Lynn Jones

Modern History Press

Ann Arbor, MI

More Confessions of a Trauma Junkie: My Life as a Nurse Paramedic; Folie à Deux, 2nd Edition
Copyright © 2012, 2021 by Sherry Lynn Jones. All Rights Reserved.

Library of Congress Cataloging-in-Publication Data

Names: Mayo, Sherry Jones, 1955- author.
Title: More confessions of a trauma junkie : my life as a nurse paramedic : folie à deux / Sherry Lynn Jones.
Other titles: Confessions of a trauma junkie
Description: 2nd edition. | Ann Arbor, MI : Modern History Press, [2021] | Revision of: Confessions of a trauma junkie. 2009. | Includes bibliographical references and index. | Summary: "Southeast Michigan nurse Sherry Lynn Jones portrays events in her career in emergency medicine including venues such as Civil Air Patrol (CAP), hospital emergency rooms, Emergency Medical Services (EMS), prisons, and crisis/disaster responses such as Hurricane Katrina. Emphasis on the need for peer-support and self-care for all types of responders"-- Provided by publisher.
Identifiers: LCCN 2020058339 (print) | LCCN 2020058340 (ebook) | ISBN 9781615995530 (paperback) | ISBN 9781615995547 (hardcover) | ISBN 9781615995554 (epub)
Subjects: LCSH: Mayo, Sherry Jones, 1955- | Nurses--Biography. | Emergency medical technicians--Biography. | Emergency nursing--Biography.
Classification: LCC RT120.E4 M345 2021 (print) | LCC RT120.E4 (ebook) | DDC 610.73092 [B]--dc23
LC record available at https://lccn.loc.gov/2020058339
LC ebook record available at https://lccn.loc.gov/2020058340

Distributed by Ingram (USA/CAN), Bertram's Books (UK/EU)

Published by Modern History Press,
5145 Pontiac Trail
Ann Arbor, MI 48105

www.ModernHistoryPress.com   Tollfree 888-761-6268
info@ModernHistoryPress.com   Fax 734-663-6681
Look for audiobook editions at Audible.com and iTunes.

Dedicated to Mama and Dad,
Who taught me duty, honor, and respect,
And that second to God,
Family is everything.

La famiglia è tutto

Table of Contents

Foreword	iii
Preface: Our Emergency Services Subculture and "It"	vii
Part I – ER and EMS: Inside the Double Doors	1
I'm Sorry... Could You Repeat That?	1
Advice to an ER Newbie	12
Rated X (and Eww!): Not for Everyone	16
Part II – When Reality is Not Shared	29
Captain Hersler	30
Myths, Medicine, and Mocking	35
Possession is $9/10^{ths}$ of the Psyche	43
Mental Notes on Paper	47
Part III – Both Sides of the Gurney	59
Stepping through Alice's Mirror	59
Some of My Favorite Things	66
Honey, TJ, and Caesar	82
Part IV – Ah... Memories	89
Bowling, Anyone?	90
Just Between Friends	93
When Not to Work a Code	104
Part V – Crisis and Disaster Response	109
Getting the Call	109
The Teacher is In ...	112
Post-Katrina: A (Military) Responder's Recollection	117
Glossary	131
References	139
About the Author	141
Index	143

Foreword

I have the honor of introducing this life-lived book, representing how many of us within the Emergency Service (ES) professions wade through our careers and lives. We see a different side of life from our first call of the day, whether in the field, the communications center, the ER, or in-flight on a chopper responding to the unknown. We see more in a day than most will ever see in a lifetime, yet we keep on doing it; this book is a testament to how and why we are able to do what we do. Sherry expresses in simple, easy-to-read terms the highs and lows within our days. Indeed; this book can be applied to all lives and all jobs, and once you read it, you will understand why I highly recommend reading it from its dedication to the very end.

I thank Sherry for the care and honor she bestows upon our families, appreciating that the most important family is the one we go home to after work. The significance and need for family awareness, so often overlooked, is entrenched within the pages of this book. Sherry paints a picture of the necessity of hearing what is said, and also the more essential and sometimes difficult task of closely listening for, and hearing, what is not said. She brings this out succinctly when speaking of being at home with our loved ones and being at work with our second (work) family, and how we live balancing an emotional house of cards on a sand foundation. We need to be aware of what our loved one/partner at home or work is saying, not saying, how he or she demonstrates thoughts and feelings, and if those behaviors are atypical for the personality we feel we know.

One of my greatest takes from Sherry's latest book is the viewpoint of her personal familiarity as an Emergency Service professional. It is as if she is looking through a prism because Sherry gives a perspective viewed through the spectrum of an entire life filled with so many colors and dimensions, telling exactly how an Emergency Service professional lives. It brings us to the highs we are blessed with throughout our careers, and the hilarity of some of the silliness in all our lives while taking us to that other spectrum, where the unknown is alive, well and as always, unexpected.

We can never be prepared for all emergencies regardless of how much we train. Sherry brings out how we cannot train for everything and we *must* always have a backup plan. Sometimes even those backup plans are not successful, but we can always say we tried our best! Since Sherry's first wonderful book, *Confessions of a Trauma Junkie* (2009), just look what this tiny place we call home, (the world), has gone through, like massive earthquakes in Haiti (2010) and Japan (2011). Whether it is the wrath of natural disasters or wars (because humankind does not learn from history), we need to work out what we could have done differently to help.

I am empowered by reading Sherry's book as no doubt you will be too, regardless of what you do professionally; it is a book about true life and living. It is both an introspective view as well as a stark reminder of the importance of being there for the ES professional, ready to deliver caring, non-judgmental thoughts and making the time to listen. We (ES) are always the last to ask for help, yet we will always be on the frontlines for others. Sherry captures and relates sights and smells of past traumas addressed (or not) and the silliness of all humankind within the covers of this book.

What Sherry Jones has once again taken to the reader (laypersons or in related fields) may seem like a moment in time yet has enveloped an entire lifetime, a career, a love, a day in the life of us the "street people." She speaks for the true Trauma Junkies of the world who have confessions as yet untold and careers with more to learn. My thanks go to Sherry for this wonderful book written about those of us who have been given the honor to care for those in need. My thanks and blessings to all of my global brothers and sisters both in uniform or in training who share the same creed of caring we all share within the Emergency Service professions.

Neal E. Braverman - Lt. Boston EMS (Ret.)
Co-Founder-Boston EMS Peer Support Team,
President Emeritus- The Metro-Boston CISM Team,

Founder - The *RESCUE* Network International
(Retired Emergency Services Critical & Continual
Understanding and Empathy Support Network)

Preface: Our Emergency Services Subculture and "It"

We in emergency services—EMS, law enforcement, trauma nurses, firefighters, military, paramilitary, corrections, and public health—have formed a bond closer than most families. With that bond are many universal understandings. We think we are superheroes as we run toward disaster instead of away from it, trying to protect total strangers from the ravages of illness, injury, harm, or self-inflicted wounds and drama.

Imposing ourselves into various crises, we try to apply all types of salves to soothe and heal, sometimes unsuccessfully, and we are not always able to keep from catching "it." We think that we are above "it" and "its" effects. Yet, like a microscopic invader of our mental and emotional health and well-being, "it" gets inside and transforms us so insidiously that we may not notice.

"It" is our enemy.

Like a pandemic worthy of rock-star-concert fund-raising, "it" has invaded us in ways we cannot describe. I suppose "it" could bear the label of stress, a simple word that deceivably carries far more pathologic potential than six simple letters communicate. Celebrity medical professionals, psychologists, and the latest reality TV shows explain and excuse erratic and sometimes illegal behaviors, offering this one dismissive word, stress, as an explanation for pretty much everything.

"It" lurks in every moment of this special group, my group, who share the delusion that we who run toward Hell instead of away from it are above the danger. Our shared delusion may be that we are physically and emotionally exempt from the ravages of stressors because of our uniforms and mental fortitude. We have developed an impenetrable, indiscernible, camouflage-colored Trauma Armor.

We rationalize that we are *safe*, although we know that safety is merely a fantasy. There is no safe place. We hold tightly to our vests, an illusion of control about things that go bump in the night. Please do not try to remove it, lest we crumble.

This book is a compilation of experiences between me and my brothers and sisters in uniform. These tales come from folks who work in emergency and disaster response situations, medical and mental health, paid and volunteer, coming from all over the country, and spanning several decades. Names have been changed to protect the innocent (or guilty). Because EMS and ER folks commonly work for multiple agencies, any attempt to identify specific patients is quite futile.

The facts and locations of each story have changed significantly to protect patient privacy. Dare I say the Health Insurance Portability and Accountability Act (HIPAA)? More formally this 1996 law includes the Privacy Rule, which strictly prohibits disclosing identifying particulars.

Those who read my mental meanderings know I am a spiritual being in a physical body, acknowledging a universe created and managed by a higher power. I recognize there are gifts bestowed by that power, and that by myself, I am simply a collection of energy and matter. I am also my mother's child, a product of her wisdom, kindness, generosity, and heritage.

As long as I have my family, "It" will never win, because I have a safe place to go. Family is the reason I am alive, the reason I found my voice, and the reason I tell these stories. Sometimes family members are the *source* of the stories, but so far, no one has required therapy. Take from this minor self-revelation the greatest survival mechanism: support systems.

Having extraordinary people whispering encouragement and walking with you through the hard stuff is incredibly important. My support systems include a wingman from Chicago, and adopted brothers from all over the U.S. Thanks to all, including big sister Nonie who stands in Mama's place, Topher, and Missy.

Learning about the emotional aftermath of trauma comes from the International Critical Incident Stress Foundation (ICISF) through Jeffrey T. Mitchell, Ph.D., CTS; George S. Everly, Jr., Ph.D., FAPM, CTS; Victor Welzant, PsyD, and Dennis Potter, LMSW, FAAETS. They are the teachers who preach the message of Critical Incident Stress Management (CISM) and provide proven methods of preparation and response thwarting the

Boogie Man. These are present-day slayers of real and imagined dragons. Thank you for having the courage to peek into the protected emotional reality of emergency services workers. Our world is a place where our feelings remain defensively shrouded behind a labyrinth of gallows humor, too much caffeine, and closed ranks, lest "it" should find us.

Truth: we are fallible. We are human. Through this book, I want you to know what we think and feel in the course of our day, our duties, our lives, and how we bring you home with us. If we seem emotionally detached, it could be that you have touched our hearts, and we are trying to keep a professional distance to continue working.

On the anniversary of my Dad's death, daughter Missy wrote, "It's not that I forgot the date, Gramps, it's that I choose not to remember when you left." That is how we often deal with things; we do not talk about them. We need to talk *more* about what is inside, but our coping mechanisms include an extremely well developed stiff upper lip. If you remind us of something or someone in our own lives, we will probably pull even deeper inside to protect ourselves, to intellectualize, to keep functioning.

We have families, we have children, we suffer physical ailments, we know what pain feels like, and we bear scars (both emotional and physical). We do not share those things with you because on the job, they are of no consequence. We leave our personal lives and complaints, to the best of our ability, at home. When we are on the job, all that matters is *you*.

This second edition of More Confessions brings you a retrospective with the 20/20 "If I knew then what I know now" viewpoint. My first observation is the wisdom in Missy's reframing of her grandfather's death. She did not bury the pain; she learned to remember and celebrate the good things. She worked through the pain, not around it. There will be tears and laughter because the processing of loss is a lifelong thing.

We don't live in the past, yet many emergency responders and ER folks still hold tight to the peers with whom they developed deep relationships "back in the day," and welcome those with similar experiences they meet in the present. Social media provides a forum for meeting, reminiscing, supporting, sometimes disagreeing, and occasionally judging. The revolving doors continue to swing as we peek back. If only we could *go* back. How different everything would be! Or would it?

Part I

ER and EMS:
Inside the Double Doors

Patients say things to us that are far better than comedy writers might ever imagine. When we try to repeat those stories, we may lose a little in translation, but clearly, patients do not always speak the same language as health care workers. Sometimes the health care providers themselves botch communications in creative ways. Whether the double doors lead to the back of an ambulance or the entrance to the Emergency Room, we all share "say what?" moments that are confounding at the time but provide fodder worth sharing with our coworkers after the call (or ER care) is over. Here are a few conversations between people who thought they were on the same page only to find they were not even in the same book.

I'm Sorry... Could You Repeat That?

"Is that going to hurt?" I am inches from your arm with a sharp needle that is about to pierce your skin and enter your vein. There are nerve endings that are invisible to the naked eye; we know they are in there, but we cannot see them. Sometimes we hit one, and sometimes we go through the vein (especially if you jump, wiggle, flail your arms, and scream). We are not trying to cause harm, and a fast IV is better for both of us.

I am very good with needles, and I can get an IV where other folks might not even attempt it. After 11 years in a Detroit Trauma Center, I can get blood out of a rock, and almost all past coworkers have at some point asked me to get an IV for them, including the resident physicians. I will pull the skin tight, enter with lightning-fast speed, draw the blood, and have the line connected and taped down before you can say ouch, even if it is in your foot. I *am* that good, but no matter how high my skill level, I am stabbing you with a sharp instrument.

Yes, it is going to hurt.

~ ~ ~

Mikey* began working in EMS long before me and remained long after I left; he is still running around in ambulances, scraping people up off the roads and coming into their lives at the most inopportune moments. Mikey says he has more "Huh?"—"Say what?" incidents than he cares to admit. Maybe it is a sign of the times.

On his first call of the day, Mikey responded to an unknown medical complaint in an apartment building. Sitting on the edge of her bed was a female patient who burst into tears when she saw Mikey walk into her room. When asked what was wrong, the patient responded that she had double vision and could see two Mikeys standing in front of her. Trying not to laugh at what struck him as a comical visual image of sudden personal cloning, Mikey and the patient concluded that a trip to the hospital was probably in order.

As Mikey and his partner were tucking the patient into the stretcher with fashionable EMS blankets, there was a sudden knock on the door. The patient asked Mikey to see who was there. When Mikey stuck his head out the door, a "frumpy little man" who lived down the hall looked up at Mikey and demanded to know what was going on.

Temporarily dumbfounded, Mikey repeated, "What is going on?" Most folks who see two uniformed men wearing radios, carrying a medical jump kit, pushing a gurney piled with heart monitor, equipment, and an oxygen tank, can figure out what is going on without a lot of explanation. To his credit, Mikey gathered every bit of self-control and resisted the temptation to utter what he wanted to say. He replied to this unknown visitor who wanted an explanation for the 911 emergency: "Sir, we are having a Tupperware party, and were just about to start burping our lids. Want to join us?"

---

* Some names are changed; the first time a pseudonym appears in the text, it is marked with an asterisk

~ ~ ~

ER tech Campbell* relates a triage moment representing many confounding exchanges with patients as staff tried to determine the patient's chief complaint. A young man walked up to the desk and told Campbell the patient's girlfriend had "burned" him. Campbell asked if it was with water, oil, lighter fluid, curling iron, the stove? The man shook his head repeatedly while looking down, repeating, "My girlfriend *burned* me!"

Becoming exasperated, Campbell thought if she could not determine the mechanism of injury (cause of the burn), perhaps she could establish the location of the injury. "Sir, can you tell me *where* you were burned?" Without raising his eyes, the young man said, "On my Hmm-Hmm," and the skies opened to rain down realization on this normally perceptive young woman. The fellow was trying to obtain treatment for the sexually transmitted disease that he believed his girlfriend gave him.

~ ~ ~

A local firefighter/paramedic tells me about a conversation witnessed between his partner Chris* and a patient. A 30-year-old healthy female, without any medical history, taking no medications, complained of chest pain. She insisted she had a heart attack. The advanced critical care paramedics connected the woman to a 12-lead EKG monitor (same as in the emergency room), assessed her vital signs, and tried to reassure her that she did not have a heart attack.

Incensed, the woman insisted, "I AM having a heart attack! I am a nursing student, so I KNOW what a heart attack feels like!" As the medic in charge of her care, Chris engaged mouth before brain, telling the patient, "Yeah, well... I took a cooking class once, but that doesn't make me a chef."

~ ~ ~

Medic Jeff S. traveled by ambulance to a home in a large mid-Michigan city, dispatched for a patient who could not "make water." Upon arrival, Jeff attempted to obtain the chief complaint from the patient's wife, who insistently repeated the same words without clarification. Although Jeff rephrased the question several times, he always got the same answer, and still had no idea what the wife was trying to convey.

Thinking literally, Jeff tells me, "I had no clue. I thought, "What is she talking about? You turn on the faucet to make water." During his brief assessment, Jeff discovered that the patient could not *pee*.

~ ~ ~

I worked with Jeff S. for many years in a very small town. He was an EMS guru from the big city, responsible for organizing and stocking our ambulances. If Jeff was the medic in charge and attending a patient during transport, more often than not, he declared that we did not carry bedpans in the ambulance.

One expected sequela of a motor vehicle crash (MVC), especially with females, is the sudden urge to void (pee, urinate, or "make water"). MVC patients routinely find themselves sporting a cervical (neck) collar, secured with straps to a long backboard to protect the spine (neck and back). Maneuvering a patient onto a bedpan in a moving ambulance is unsafe. If someone is unstable and must urinate, we have told them to go ahead and relieve themselves, and we will clean it up later. Better to be a little wet than permanently disabled.

On a particularly long transport of a stable patient, I searched through the storage compartment under the ambulance's bench seat for a blanket, finding a well-hidden but familiar pink plastic basin. Females usually cannot ride five hours without emptying their bladders, so I retrieved the bedpan for our patient. The nurse in me assisted the patient and felt quite satisfied at providing one small comfort to a very grateful woman. As I tried to place the bedpan on the floor of the moving ambulance while preventing the generous contents from sloshing all over our immaculately clean floor, I understood why Jeff preferred not to provide bedpan service. Score at the end of the transport, *Jeff: 1, Rookie: 0.*

~ ~ ~

Mike A. relays a conversation between himself and an alleged seizure patient at the local jail. Seizure is a common complaint from inmates activating their medical "get out of jail free" card, so one never knows what to expect. Many who find themselves incarcerated prefer the warm blanket, footies, turkey sandwich, juice, and friendly nurse in the emergency room to a cold jail cell and often-colder demeanor of attending officers. In short, many medical complaints from jailed complainants have no sound physiological basis.

This particular exchange is truly a head-scratcher, worthy of repeating, and provides sound social commentary. In the process of medically assessing the jailed "seizure" patient, Mike came across multiple marks on the patient's skin indicating a history of IVDA (intravenous drug use).

Mike: "Ma'am, what are these needle marks from?"
Patient: "Heroin."
Mike: "How much do you use?"
Patient: "I spend $800 a month on it."
Mike: "Wow, that's a lot; you must have a good job."
Patient: "No, I spend my Social Security check on it."
Mike: "You're very young. Why do you get Social Security?"
Patient: "I'm disabled."
Mike: "Why are you disabled?"
Patient: "I'm chemically dependent [on Heroin]."
Your tax dollars at work.

~ ~ ~

Laurie S.W. is an amazing nurse. She has a no-nonsense demeanor that required some personal adjustment and adaptation from me when I started working in my first trauma center. Once I understood Laurie, we had the type of verbal exchanges that might seem hostile, but they were all in good fun and helped us deflect stress. The good-natured bantering also helped us to keep from expressing our frustrations in negative and unproductive ways, like toward the patients or staff who sent us teetering too close to the proverbial emotional "edge."

Years ago, patient names were neither disguised nor confidential. To organize ourselves in the ER, we wrote the patient's last names on a dry-erase board. One afternoon when things were not so busy and the patients, who had nothing to do but wait for tests and watch the staff buzz around, noticed the odd exchanges between Laurie and me. Every half hour or so, Laurie or I would point to the dry erase board, and the other would acknowledge, often with a laugh, protruding tongue, or a hand gesture involving limited numbers of fingers.

One family in the corner of the room had the best view and called me over, expecting an explanation of our shenanigans. Because I had been interacting with those folks for several hours, I knew they had a sense of humor and might appreciate the private joke.

Laurie had written "STFU" on the dry erase board in large letters. Unable to stand the suspense any longer, the family had to know what the acronym meant, and I was happy to share the secret. STFU is, as most folks know in this day of texting acronyms, an obscene translation of the phrase, "Shut The Front Door!"

Can you feel the love?

~ ~ ~

Serina L. rendered me speechless with something I had never considered before (and they say there is nothing new under the sun). A young female seen in the ER for abdominal pain had a normal workup, which included a pregnancy test. Not surprisingly, the pregnancy test was positive.

When told by the nurse that she was pregnant, the patient—who was completely shocked and baffled—replied, "But I thought you couldn't GET pregnant when you had Chlamydia!" Are sexually transmitted diseases a form of birth control? I must have missed that day in nursing school.

~ ~ ~

When a nurse or medic administers narcotics without using the entire vial of medication, another staff member must corroborate the appropriate disposal of the remainder of the vial. We call the disposition of excess narcotics "wasting." In the ER, you may hear the summons for a staff member to come to the locked medication room as "nurse to the med room for a waste, please."

Sometimes the harried nurses spew twisted utterances, providing cause for a double-take. Overheard in a large city ER, where drug abuse and stress levels were both quite high: "Nurse to the med room to get wasted, please!" Oops. Do-over?

"Do you want to see this?" is a question posed by patients who are sure you will not believe the color or consistency of what they have produced from their nose, rectum, stomach, or elsewhere. We do not want to see. We believe your mastery of language is sufficient to describe the suspicious emergence, thank you.

We will even put your vibrant and animated description in quotes throughout our nurses' notes to assure a relatively precise accounting of what ails you, and from where it came. Please do not fish it out of the toilet so we can send it to the lab. We can only use hospital-gathered specimens. I always advise patients to leave whatever they have gathered at home.

Gallows humor prevented me from following that advice. Yes, I did this. Yes, it was awesome.

After returning from a teaching deployment in Alaska, I paid a visit to my internal medicine doc, Seth P. I had known Seth and his then-wife, Monica, all through their residencies. Seth was quite a prankster, and once whispered, as we stood at the foot of an unconscious patient's bed, that he and Monica had separated. When I told Monica I was sorry to hear the news and explained the conversation, she rolled her eyes and said, "That's OK, I tell people he's dead."

Paybacks are Heck, Bubba.

I sat across from Seth at his office desk, uncomfortably clutching a paper bag. Apologizing, I told Seth I knew how unpleasant samples could be regardless of our professionalism, but I had something to show him. I slowly opened the bag, revealing a ratty paper-towel-wrapped item. Spending a few moments explaining that this was something I had never seen before, I slowly pulled the wrapping from around the medical specimen cup. Inside the clear cup, Seth and I could both see something small wrapped in crumpled toilet paper.

Preparing Seth further, I said, "This is a stool sample. I carried it back from Alaska for you." I placed the cup in front of him. Scrunching his face in preparation for something completely disgusting, Seth asked if he needed gloves. I shrugged and watched him gingerly unscrew the cap of the specimen cup. He hesitated, so I took the cup from him, dumping the contents onto his desk; he jumped.

Pulling the tissue from around the "specimen," I revealed the object carried back from Alaska. The cup held a thumb-sized glass jar marked "Stool Sample" and contained a miniature wooden *stool* (the four-legged variety used to sit upon).

Bazinga!

~ ~ ~

Triage nurses hear a good number of intriguing stories, and sometimes generally mundane complaints produce the most interesting results. A woman presents to triage complaining of impending labor. However, because she doesn't have an obstetrician or a positive pregnancy test, and she doesn't look pregnant, she may not be rushed to the labor and delivery suites. Patients fitting this description come to the triage desk quite often and with predictable results. They usually suffer from some female problem, go home with a prescription for Motrin, and live happily ever after.

A nurse friend of mine tells about the day this normally uninteresting type of complaint had an O. Henry (or Edgar Allen Poe) ending. The triage nurse generated the appropriate chart, and escorted the patient to a "girl room" (breakaway bed with stirrups). The nurse showed the woman a sterile urine cup, asking her to provide a sample, and then put the cup on the bedside table.

The patient's primary nurse ran the urine test. The patient was not pregnant. Following protocol, the nurse set the patient up for a pelvic exam and waited for the doctor. When the doc exposed the woman's private parts, he saw the labia closed by three large safety pins, with what appeared to be remnants of raw chicken protruding between the pins.

I have no further comment.

~ ~ ~

Dee S. and I worked together in a 75-bed city Trauma Center, with, on a busy day, more than 100 patients. Some weeks we ran out of the rolling multi-fold dividers intended to provide visual barriers between patients doubled together in single rooms.

Trying to maintain appropriate patient care with too many patients and too little privacy challenged us daily. Dee was city savvy and saw the comical side of everything, often sprinkling snippets of humor like anti-stress fairy dust.

Assisting patients with transportation was one of Dee's duties. Some folks arrived via ambulance, and legitimately had no way to return home. Other times, folks wanted the "free" ride, insisting they had no family or friends, denying the multiple visitors at their bedside (or asleep in the lobby) during their stay. The patients who knew and regularly used the "free ride" system often proclaimed, "And don't you give me no bus voucher, I know you can order me a cab. I want my cab. I don't ride no bus."

Dee relates a "head shaking, what the heck?" moment.

A young male in his twenties walked into the ER, through the metal detectors, and up to the triage desk where Dee met him. The young man told Dee he'd visited the ER yesterday, and though he had requested bus tickets home yesterday, he did not get them... yesterday. He wanted them now.

Dee: "How did you get home [yesterday]?"

Patient: "I walked."

Dee: "How did you get here today?"

Patient: "I walked"

Dee: "So you walked back here today just to get bus tickets to go back home?"

Patient: (silence).

~ ~ ~

Paramedic Schultz tells me that he spends a lot of time teaching EMT students at the Mayo Clinic. Duly impressed, I listened intently for words of wisdom from this excellent medic who had seen it all. One day he was about to deliver another profound pearl of wisdom. As I leaned in to catch this new tidbit, Schultz informed me of "The three Ps of Emergency Medicine." Expecting a new acronym or algorithm, I was surprised to hear the explanation. Unfortunately, for me, I asked him to repeat it—twice—before understanding that he said, "Pee, Poop, and Puke."

~ ~ ~

We medics never know what we might face when responding to a call. Our dispatcher has accurately recorded and reiterated to us all the information provided, yet somehow the story changes between that initial 911 request and our arrival. We are sometimes lulled into a sense of sameness, and then out of nowhere we meet someone like Millie.*

Millie was a lonely woman in her mid-fifties who lived on the seventh floor of a cramped inner-city apartment building. Summers were hotter in the city, and the evening darkness did not provide much of a break. Following weeks of unforgiving heat, in a building where air conditioning consisted of wobbly department store fans propped clumsily in bedroom windows, desperate folks like Millie called 911 for a free trip to an air-conditioned ER.

Complaints used most often were chest pain and difficulty breathing. Callers knew priority complaints ensured priority responses. Lesser complaints meant a "free" EMS (community taxi) ride but did not guarantee going straight into an ER bed.

Because Millie chose chest pain as her complaint on this hot, humid, summer afternoon, we were obligated to assume a legitimate cardiac problem until proven otherwise. We pulled out our drug box, jump kit, oxygen, and cardiac monitor, piling them on the stretcher.

Fortunately, one of the elevators worked, and we soon arrived at Millie's door. When we knocked on the closed and latched door, we heard "just a minute," followed by the sound of multiple locks opening, and then a rapid "thump, thump, thump" as Millie ran away. The door creaked as we pushed it open, and we heard a voice bellowing, "I'm in the bedroom!"

I am sorry, could you please repeat that?

We followed the moans to where Millie lay thrashing about on her bed. She made good time running from the front door to her position in the bedroom, but thrashing was far more dramatic than standing at the door, so we understood.

Conveniently, Millie's unbuttoned blouse and no bra provided easy access for EKG lead placement. As we prepared Millie for transport (after noting her perfect EKG and lack of medical history except for gross obesity), we gave each other a knowing look as the bigger picture flowed over us.

Our backs can expect that anyone over 350 pounds will not walk when we arrive, even though they were almost running moments before. Often someone without a significant medical history, taking no cardiac medications, will complain of chest pain. We had seen many times the lack of decorum by patients who thought nothing of presenting semi-nude to total strangers. None of these things entered our minds.

That day, we were not rolling our eyes at the umpteenth call from a building without air conditioning on a hot summer day. We recognized and wordlessly acknowledged to one another, "Yes, there is a God." Because despite completely different views between the patient and ourselves about what constitutes a medical emergency, we accepted a divine intervention. On this day, with this patient, and on this call, the elevator was working.

~ ~ ~

John B., a Physician's Assistant (PA) with whom I enjoyed a brief working relationship in an extremely busy Las Vegas ER, relays a poignant example of why ER-Speak and People-Speak are often diametrically opposite in nature and understanding. John is a fabulous and unflappable PA who takes the time to make sure patients understand their test results, often using non-clinical terms. I am quite sure John stifled a giggle at the following exchange. John said, "I told a patient, "The wet reading on your x-rays didn't show any fractures." The patient, looking confused, asked, 'Should we wait till it gets dry?'"

Ba-dum-bum-ching! Thank you, and please remember to tip your waitperson.

~ ~ ~

Big Ed was an imposing figure who sat me down for a "come to Jesus" meeting shortly after I started my ER RN job in a large Midwestern Trauma Center. We did not know each other, and even though I felt somewhat capable as a paramedic turned RN, ER Tech Ed let me know that I was green. He did not trust me, and I would have to prove myself. It seemed harsh, but I soon understood the level of trust necessary not only for patient care but also for personal safety. It was a rough city and a tough place to work for anyone lacking "street cred." What Ed and most folks I worked with did not know was that I was born and raised in Detroit (and its suburbs), spending several years working EMS on the city streets.

As a former bouncer, Big Ed was better to have around than an armed security officer. Sustaining injuries from a patient or family member was part of the job unless you had Ed on your team. This story shares Ed's advice to anyone working in a challenging inner-city ER from the perspective of a boy from the 'hood, born and raised in Detroit, Michigan. Ed was an Emergency Room technician for eight years before moving on to other endeavors. He now lives in South Dakota, working in the firearms industry. How appropriate.

Advice to an ER Newbie

Written with (and from the perspective of) Ed Dunnigan, ERT.

If you work in an ER, eventually you will encounter patients. Patients are the people who come in a seemingly endless stream seeking medical attention for whatever ails them, descending upon the ER for complaints ranging from minor cuts to major strokes.

Newbie ER employees commonly approach these patients intending to spread goodwill through healing, which is not so easy. The majority of those coming to the ER consider their visit to the hospital a necessary evil. They come because they are in pain, sick, lonely, bleeding, addicted to something, withdrawing from something, high on something, drunk, giving birth, or dying. Patient attitudes vary from anxiety to hostility. One cannot always assuage those emotions.

The first hurdle to overcome in the ER environment is learning not to take anything personally. In any large city, the majority of the people who frequent the local ER almost certainly wear a label of "The Underclass." Most of these folks spend their lifetimes in poverty. Many have no hope, are generally uneducated or undereducated, often live in single-parent homes, and believe everything is someone else's fault.

To survive, the ER newbie must understand that sometimes he and the majority of inner-city patients come from opposing worldviews. Retiring at age fourteen, completing formal education in the seventh grade, and spending days in a drug-filled haze conceiving illegitimate children may not reflect a life of goal setting and achievements, but that is the life known by many inner-city residents.

They learn from one generation to the next that they bear no responsibility for their lifestyle. Had others not oppressed them and refused them the same opportunities and advantages of the privileged class, they would be affluent too. Trying to educate them that anyone can rise above circumstances and step away from victim status falls on deaf ears, eliciting charges of elitism. Many live by government handouts, seeing those entitlements as their right.

I offer this personal perspective to prepare newbies for the baggage that accompanies those attitudes, which I theorize as the "Prison Affectation." In prison, the slightest insult results in violence. Something as simple as a hard look can get people injured or killed. In inner-city neighborhoods, hardened and violent ex-cons are common. Often, they bring the attitude and temperament, a learned-behavioral method of survival, out onto the streets with them.

Young people emulate these role models. If someone "disses" those folks (street vernacular for "disrespects"), violence ensues, and retaliation follows. It is precisely this attitude that will keep inner-city ERs running 24/7.

The newbie must learn to communicate without being condescending or insulting, a fine line discerned through experience. Learning the vernacular of the region is imperative. I was lucky because the ER where I worked the midnight shift for so many years was very near the neighborhood where I grew up. My theories stem from experience, lest anyone question my position. I lived it. I understood the patients and their families, and often assumed the role of "interpreter" for some of my co-workers.

Listening to a drunk, high, gang-banger tell what happened to him, using street language, and then repeating his story in The King's English so that the doctor from wherever can understand, is a surreal experience.

Gang-banger: "Yo, man! I was strollin' through the 'hood, mindin' my own bidness, when this hoopty roll up on the set and these mutha f—s start bustin' caps! I was breakin' wide when somethin' hit me. I dove behind my boy's crib 'til five-o pulled up!"

Translation: "I was walking down the street when a car pulled up, and the occupants started shooting at me. I was running when I felt the bullet hit me. I hid behind my friend's house until the police arrived."

The patients and their families in these situations are often loud and vulgar. I have heard it said that profanity is simply a weak mind attempting to express itself forcefully. Remember newbie: the people you deal with have neither the vocabulary nor the sophistication to articulate their thoughts or feelings as you may desire.

Instead, they curse when they wish to be emphatic, they increase their volume when they wish to drive home a point. This is NOT to say that these folks are stupid. They are simply attempting to communicate within the limitations of their education and experience. You, as the professional, must learn to listen beyond the words and hear what they are saying.

How does one accomplish this necessary connection? Remove your ego from the equation. The yelling and the profanity reflect a learned method of dealing with the world. No personal indictment exists.

Many of these folks live within the bureaucratic nightmare of whatever welfare agency handles their case. Dealing with bureaucracy reinforces their particular brand of assertiveness (rude and obnoxious behavior) as the only method effective to assure desired results.

Stay calm. Be attentive. Be aware of what the patient is DOING as well as what they are saying (situational awareness) for your safety and survival.

The important thing for you to remember, newbie, is that although others come from a background that is probably very different from yours, they are entitled to all of the respect that you afford anyone else. Dealing with them as an equal will put them at ease and make your job much easier.

We are fast becoming a global society, and cultural awareness includes knowing you are not the only one. Your way is not the only way. Tolerance begins here and now.

~ ~ ~

This book is intentionally lacking in expletives and racy stories out of respect for the wide range of readers. During relaying truthful exchanges between the public and emergency services folks, and sharing how we feel about them, sometimes things can get a little spicy. Or weird and icky. To allow you an honest exploration into our day, we will admit to having certain calls and patients that make us cringe, blush, stifle giggles, gag, and sometimes flee. There are also times that we must briefly excuse ourselves from the public. If we do not, our professionalism may crumble under the enormous and probably tearful belly laugh that emanates from deep inside us, a place beyond our conscious control.

There are also occasions when the mechanism of injury or source of a medical complaint occurs during intimate moments. We try especially hard to remain professional, sensitive, caring, and non-judgmental. These are the things that might make entertaining television. However, after viewing the tasteless and inane fodder that creates reality TV celebrities for all the wrong reasons, the documentation in this section is quite tame.

Rated X (and Eww!): Not for Everyone

Folks have heart attacks at the most inopportune moments. Facing a crew of uniformed police officers, paramedics, firefighters, and anyone else who responds in a professional capacity to a 911 call can make an emotional situation exponentially more uncomfortable. One such call came over the paging system from central dispatch that was vague enough to indicate that all hands should respond, as a two-person crew might be insufficient. An "unresponsive" patient usually did not have a pulse or respirations.

A volunteer EMT-trainee named Randy[*] worked with an ambulance service in a very small town some years back. He had a pager that was on and accessible every waking moment. If the call promised to provide learning opportunities, or if crews required extra hands, Randy was to respond to the call's location from home. This particular day, a few hours after lunch, Randy was at the station when the dispatcher sent his Alpha (Advanced

Life Support/ALS) unit to a private home for an unresponsive male in his late fifties.

The patient slouched in a wheelchair with a frantic female standing next to him, dressed in something that could pass euphemistically for a negligee. Several of the responders attended to the clinical needs of the patient, who was in full cardio-pulmonary arrest. One of the medics tried to get information from the woman: medical history, medications, and allergies. When the medic questioning the woman tried to find out what the patient was doing immediately before slumping over in his wheelchair, the woman, who had composed herself enough to answer questions, suddenly became quite uncomfortable.

Struggling for words, the best the woman could muster in the way of explanation was that she was "loving on him" when the patient stopped breathing. Not sure that he had heard her correctly, the medic asked for clarification. The woman shrieked the same words again at the top of her voice. The proverbial light bulb popped on above Randy's head, and slightly embarrassed, he quickly excused himself to accompany the rest of the crew in the ambulance. I'll have more to share about "Uncle Randy" in later chapters.

~ ~ ~

Sometimes people do things they might not have attempted if compliant with their prescribed medications, and "in their right mind." Jay* tells me about an embarrassing situation for a young man that became a life-threatening situation, not something one sees every day. What completely puzzles me is the extent to which people will go for self-gratification, and how complex the procedures, especially when technology of any kind is involved. Let me relay Jay's story without going into too much graphic detail.

A young man took a safety pin and poked a hole in his scrotum large enough to accommodate a rubber tube connected to a small air compressor. Pushing the tube far enough into his scrotum to seal the entry hole, the fellow turned the compressor on for about 3-4 minutes, successfully forcing enough air into his system to infiltrate below his skin from his neck down to his toes. Pressing on his skin resulted in a kind of popping sensation, rendering him into what Jay described human bubble wrap. We call it subcutaneous emphysema, like pressing on Rice Krispies.® The patient called it doggone painful.

While staying in the hospital for several days as his body reabsorbed the insufflation (air), Jay's patient received a psych consult. Why did he do it? The short answer was "self-gratification," which Jay wryly admits gives a completely new meaning to the term "blow job."

~ ~ ~

Rick H. is an awesome ER doc who has a saucy side and quick wit, so one must listen closely to catch the subtle meaning in his deadpan delivery. Recently, Dr. Rick was in a southern state, checking out an ambulance company as a site reviewer. Rick credited the company with doing many things well, other things not so well. Dr. Rick's advice? "Let's just say that male/female squads should make sure there are no panties in the rig before an inspection." I could not have said it better.

~ ~ ~

Speaking of undergarments, as a paramedic and ER RN, I have cut clothing off more people than I can remember. Folks who come in acutely ill, or who find themselves victims of car crashes, did not get up that morning thinking, "Hmm... what shall I wear for my ER visit today?" The others, however, often give great thought to how they might present themselves. Both ends of that particular spectrum may surprise you.

Women of childbearing years who come in with lower abdominal pain, especially if pregnant, are going to receive a pelvic exam. If one is not urgently ill and can walk without effort, some attention to hygiene is a good thing. Not bathing for a week can challenge most hospital masks, and certainly most hospital personnel. Some folks think it proves they are legitimately sick if they do not wash before coming to the ER.

Dousing with perfume only exacerbates the situation. Artificial scents do not cover smells. They walk with those rancid aromas in holding hands.

While I am standing on this particular soapbox, patients and patient family members should be more considerate of others.

Perfumes are offensive, especially in mass quantities, and those who are allergic to scents can have a severe medical reaction. I have intense environmental allergies, requiring a rescue inhaler when folks wear perfumes. Patchouli can shut down my respiratory system; it should have stayed back in the 1970s and died a dignified death. On one occasion at work in the ER, I forgot my inhaler and almost stopped breathing (thank you Christopher, the magnificent pharm tech, for running an inhaler upstairs before I required intubation!).

One more thing worth mentioning at the request of my ER MD friends: you do not have to "dress for the doctor." My across the street neighbor once called and asked if I would watch one daughter while she took the other to the ER. I raced over in my sweats and slippers, only to find her putting on make-up and trying to decide which necklace to wear.

In the ER, I have seen women who come in with lingerie type undies and put their gowns on backward (opening in front), so the doc could see what was beneath the gown. Some have even lifted their blouses to expose rhinestone-studded bras (in Las Vegas), so the doctor could "see" their chest pain. Worse is no bra at all. Looking for a doctor-husband in the ER is a bad idea, and docs are not impressed with magnificent breast enhancement surgery showing "barely a scar."

Thank you very much.

~ ~ ~

Tomi, one of my favorite nurses in the Pacific Northwest, expresses her frustration with patients who find creative but unsavory (pun intended) places to hide things. One of Tomi's patients chose to use her "Va-Jay-Jay" (the professional term for vagina popularized by TV show *Grey's Anatomy*) to store drugs. Forgive me, but I believe she referred to it as a Snatch Stash. The men also have a convenient body cavity used to hide things, like drugs or weapons, called a Prison Wallet. I wish I were making this stuff up, but if I were that creative, I would email Ross Bennett and offer to write a comedy routine.

~ ~ ~

Paramedic James* recently learned a new meaning for a seemingly innocuous word: "sounding." You and I may think of "sounding" as something related to noise, but this slang term has far more masochistic undertones. According to the patient that James was attending, sounding refers to a practice related to self-gratification that involves placing foreign objects into one's urethra (down the penis). The patient had used a coat hanger, which looped through the urethra and into the bladder, where the hooked end of the hanger grasped the bladder tissue and would not let go.

Over the years, I have placed hundreds of Foley catheters through the penis into the bladder. The normal and expected reaction is men expressing extreme discomfort, usually through profanity or almost inhuman guttural sounds. I guess some things are not for everyone.

~ ~ ~

Sometimes EMS and firefighting television shows use sex to get ratings, showing a sordid side of emergency services. People do not always have intimate liaisons in hospital linen rooms or the back of an ambulance, but it does happen. In EMS, I have heard it called the "lights and sirens club" and have had several offers to join the club with a work partner, or become a member with a significant other while my partner drove the rig. I suppose that type of activity is one of many questionable coping mechanisms used by those who deal with life and death daily. I would not promote it, nor have I employed it, but since this is a confessional, I will share one personal experience.

When working in a 10-hour city car (ambulance), we did not have a station or quarters for downtime. Ready for the next call, we often sat cover (parked and waited) on some deserted corner, strategically positioning our rig between cover points. If one ambulance responded to a call, other ambulances moved to cover its areas to ensure appropriate response times for emergency (911) calls. If all of the rigs are on the west side of town and the last car available to respond is on the east side, traveling across those extra miles is problematic and could affect patient outcomes, so vehicles strategically reposition.

Because I was a "medic du jour" during nursing school (no regular assignment, part-time employee), I often had a different partner each weekend. One particular weekend I worked with a young man who had interesting conceptualizations regarding female paramedics, nurses, and redheads. I was all three. This medic thought any one person solely ringing all three bells was certainly suitable for the Halloween costume/porn perception of "Naughty Nurse Nancy." The fellow told me he was going into the back of the rig and would wait there for me.

The corner my partner (driver) had strategically selected for us to sit cover was unlit. He had backed the rig up to the edge of the woods at the far end of the parking lot. This young man, whose name I have fortunately long forgotten, fancied himself quite the Lothario. He stepped out of the ambulance and quietly entered the patient compartment from the side of the rig.

I casually pulled the heaviest nursing book from my backpack, Pediatrics as I recall, and told him that I would be staying in the front seat. As I tossed him the book, I said, "don't wait up for me; here is some light reading if you get bored." I cannot remember how long he stayed back there, likely until we got another call from dispatch. I do not think we spoke to one another again for the rest of the shift.

~ ~ ~

I must tell you about a part of our emergency services reality. Although we do not like to talk about it, ignoring the truth does not lessen its severity or effect on our lives. Please pardon any breach of etiquette, social insensitivity, or airs of elitism. I am completely honest with you about our feelings, and this is something many (if not all) of us feel at some time or another, and wish to confess.

Some patients gross us out.

We all have our frailties, and they vary between individuals. We also take great pride at being appropriately unsympathetic to our fellow workers when something bothers them and not us, reflecting our coping mechanisms and gallows humor. We are, in those circumstances, tougher, and the tough guy wins. We all want to be the tough guy.

The extent of the insensitivity is completely individualized. Whether it is funny, distracting, or "Get Over It and Get Back in the Rig," distracting depends on the circumstances. For example, a shared level of Ick and Eww comes about when called to a home with endemic cockroaches. To be more specific, when you arrive at a patient's home, and every surface seems to be moving, your Ick alarms blare. Through the dim light peeking through the newspapers taped to every window, you realize the moving carpet is a hardwood floor covered by a massive sheet of cockroaches. Ick and Eww are crawling inside your skin, and immediately you begin to itch.

Another Ick fascinating to some and worthy of running in the opposite direction to others is when maggots cover patient wounds. These are not medical maggots applied by surgeons to drain blood from post-operative wounds (pricey little buggers). These maggots occur naturally by unattended wounds that breed fly larvae in necrotic flesh. The smell is horrific, and whether in the ambulance or ER, the staff is never happy to see this type of patient. The rigs or rooms in which the patients are seen always require extra care, carefully and meticulously decontaminated after the patient goes home.

We have all been the recipient of ill-aimed bodily fluids. I escaped the diaper-less stream of the baby boy I raised (thank you, Topher), the boy he is raising (thank you, Sean), and so far the newest grandson (watch it, Andrew!), but cannot remember how many times I have worn someone else's pee. (PS, Andrew now exclusively uses the bathroom, expertly missing walls and floors.)

In the ER, those "exposures" call for a quick change of uniform. A sympathetic staff member runs to sterile supply to grab a clean set of scrubs as the peed-upon staff member limps toward the break room wearing a face of revulsion. The less sympathetic staff point and laugh.

Then there is emesis. Not many have escaped the stream of spew projecting stomach contents everywhere. EMS folks anticipate this particular Ick and Eww from patients that code, usually after eating a large ethnic meal containing copious amounts of garlic. I was the recipient of projectile vomitus once from a girl who was a member of my son's high school band. I had to act unaffected, mumbling something about "part of the job."

In the ER, sometimes that volcanic gastric eruption comes after the patient has consumed charcoal to soak up ingested poisons. Liquid charcoal does not wash out of anything, so too bad if it finds its way to your white shoes or jacket. We consider them either marks of ownership declaring one as an ER employee, or making uniforms fit for the dumpster. I have seen ER and EMS staff become so nauseated at someone else regurgitating that they vomit, or gag while fighting to swallow down what threatens to erupt all over patients. Perhaps it is empathy.

The biggest offender is mucus. God bless the ICU nurses who suction without flinching and the ER docs who replace breathing tubes coated with long, thick, green strings and globules. Sometimes the exodus is impressive (who would have thought one person could contain such copious amounts of mucus?). These patients have surely inspired Hollywood film writers.

Do we let on that we are affected? Usually not, but watch closely. If our shoulders are moving rhythmically, our mouths tightly closed with one hand pressed against them, and we are doing our best to look away, we are probably trying to keep from throwing up. Medical professionals heaving at the sight of anything our patient does or produces is very un-cool.

I remember several staff members working together, cleaning a patient withdrawing from heroin. The female patient had a continual stream of stringy, foul-smelling excrement oozing from her rectum. It took four of us to clean her, and a fifth to keep bringing clean sheets and warm washcloths. The stench traveled beyond the confines of our area, separated from the rest of the ER by a flimsy curtain.

The heap of polluted linens overflowed our soiled linen receptacle, amassing into a growing mound on the floor. As soon as we thought we had the situation under control, the dam broke again, and we started over. Looking around at my helpful staff, I noticed that one at a time, each had to turn their head and breathe into their sleeve for a moment, trying not to retch or drop out and walk away.

Have I said too much?

~ ~ ~

Here is one more confession before moving on to something lighter and less assaulting to your senses. If you are eating and reading, you may choose to skip this graphic snippet, especially if you have a good imagination. For many of us, intellectually removing ourselves from the negative visuals becomes old hat, but the assailant that defies evasion for many is smell. Death has a smell, especially if the person has been dead a long time in a warm place.

The body rots. Blowflies hover, and lay eggs, which turn to maggots. The body balloons with fluid. The skin turns black and eventually cracks open, releasing its sickening ooze.

Seasoned ES folks keep a jar of Vicks® mentholated ointment in their jump bags, and put a smear under their noses to fill scent receptors. If noses go bare and unprotected, the smell will cling for a very long time. Once you become familiar with the smell of death, the memory never leaves you.

We know other smells, too, like the smell of rotting flesh on patients who have diabetes or circulatory problems, causing tissues to necrose (die). Many patients will say, "My toe was red and painful, but now that it turned black (dead tissue), it doesn't hurt anymore. I figured I'd wait until my doctor appointment next month to check it out."

Wounds have distinctive smells, too, commonly presenting to ER nurses who assist doctors in performing I&Ds (cutting into the wound to release infected goop). The doc will stand at a safe distance, reaching from as far as the length of his arm will allow, and cut into a wound that is red, full, and teeming with pus. The nurse, unfortunately, usually stands close enough to catch (in a sterile lab container) the fountain of infected goo that forcefully springs forth. On those days, even though nothing physically touched my gowned, gloved, and masked exterior, I often felt contaminated.

We lead such glamorous lives in emergency medicine. If I called home and asked to have my robe placed in the downstairs bathroom, it was one of those Ick and Eww days. I stepped out of my shoes in the garage, dropped my uniform in the washing machine as I passed through the mudroom, and proceeded directly into the shower to wash off the funk of the day.

If you know anyone who wants to become a paramedic or nurse, you may want to share this.

POSTMORTEM

Please know that we are not laughing at you, we are trying to keep balanced, to retain our sanity, to meet the next demand. It's called gallows humor, a coping method used when people see, hear, smell, and do things they should not see, hear, smell, and do. We laugh during and after seemingly hopeless situations.

In our line of work, and in light of social justice and judgment, we keep our humor amongst ourselves. We fear that you might not understand if we shared everything. The *Trauma Junkie* anthology is a sneak peek, in short bits that you can walk away from, into how we think and feel during our experiences.

We hope you will appreciate the absurdity. Maybe you laughed at some of the writings, perhaps read them aloud to a family member or friend nearby. If so, then maybe you get it, and we thank you.

Rereading the first section of this book, I realized how much I miss the ER. I miss flying through undoable days with wings or a cape or just caffeine. Doing the impossible, then walking away unscathed, was extremely fulfilling.

The days were not always dark. Sometimes even the most horrible situations filled me with the sense that I was here for a legitimate God-given purpose in this world. Some days I cried all the way home, did not sleep, then dreamed about the bad stuff when I dozed off.

I had to put a smile on my face when I walked back into the ER the next day. Sometimes I had to find that smile five minutes after pulling the sheet over the head of a deeply-loved person because there is no time to mourn. We move on to the next, and the next, and the next.

Not mourning the losses, not taking a moment of silence, or a period to transition is the piece we are missing. Even now, learning about resilience and coping is not a big part of training beyond a short mention. Nursing and responder orientation and continuing education focus on taking care of patients and equipment, on functions and skills. Rarely do new nurses and responders have the opportunity to learn how to perform simple self-care, or to transition between work and home/home and work. The lines between personal and professional, between self and job, blur. We are often hypervigilant and fearful because we know what *might* happen.

Mindfulness tells us about living in the moment without judging the moment, a simple concept, but like most, not inherent. Studies have shown that combining mindfulness and coping strategies with task training can pair them in a way that allows responders to recall them together when needed. Until the practice of teaching coping is more prevalent, individuals will rely on their coping skills, which may be woefully lacking. Many go to the dark side to get through the tough calls, to rationalize their experiences.

In years past, the public laughed more freely at dark comedy, at those who made careers out of highlighting the most foolish realities in daily living. Today, some folks are likely to judge how wrong we are for laughing. The alternative to living in a moment with humor is to face an often horrific reality, and that can be too much to bear. If we do not push our empathy aside (and we have tons of it, or we would not be in public service), we will feel your pain. Multiply that pain by the number of patients we see a day, and it does not bode well for us. We might develop heart problems, ulcers, PTSD, depression. Oh, wait—we do.

Back then, we worried about being tough enough, strong enough. Crisis management told us that we are all human, that despite denial or supression, we have the dreaded "F" word (feelings). Over time, we learned that we all have different coping mechanisms, like gallows humor and avoidance. We learned which coping mechanisms were helpful, which were harmful.

Now, we realize an increased public and professional awareness of the damaging elements of trauma exposure. We acknowledge PTSD and suicide among emergency responders, fire, law enforcement, and corrections. Numbers are rising every day of those who have had enough and feel the only way out is closing down permanently. Hindsight always provides "woulda-coulda-shoulda." Hindsight is too late. Some of us are broken and feel there isn't enough duct tape in the world.

A paramedic on social media recently wrote about PTSD, saying we (responders) all have PTSD in some form or another. The writer asked if any of his readers had treatment or counseling. He asked if they had tried EMDR (Eye Movement Desensitization and Reprocessing), HRV (Heart Rate Variability biofeedback), ETOH (alcohol), antidepressants, antipsychotics, cannabis, aromatic oils, exercise ... or suicide. Not a complete list, not all good choices, but before you get to the last item on the writer's list, try something. Talk to someone.

Reach out.

Part II

When Reality Is Not Shared

I learned that psychosis represents a different perception involving an unshared reality. Delusions and hallucinations blur the line between those with severe mental disorders and the shared experiences of "the rest of us," we who reside on the other side of the clanging metal door for which few carry keys. I have had several psychotic experiences in my life, like when deeply engrossed in a movie or a good book. Reading transports me as I lose my sense of time and current place. I am so absorbed that if someone calls my name, they yank me back into reality. Why did you bring me back to now? I liked it there in my escape through fantasy, long-ago times, and faraway places! When presented with folks who do not see or hear what I do, who is to say my reality is the correct one? It could be a matrix matter, or a giant alien peering at us through an electron microscope as he taps impatiently with the end of a carbon nanotube. Or maybe I have a good imagination. Whether staring forward in Plato's cave or standing in bright, new sunlight, forcing an extended tortuous intellectual journey to enlightenment, sometimes things have variations of gray. Although we may not share those visions, sometimes we need to respect them, or at least show respect for the people who experience them.

Captain Hersler

Written with (and from the perspective of) Bob Tompos, EMTP

Early in my career, when the transport of these very special and interesting patients occupied the majority of my shifts, I learned that the potential to have them share my interpretation of reality was a long shot. If I was able to gather enough information to visit their parallel reality, I was often able to complete the call with a minimal amount of friction. Looking back, the psychiatric patients I transported were my most interesting calls, and I think I may have made more of a difference in those cases than on many medical runs. I know some may think I should not have bought into their delusions, but I was more concerned with getting them to comprehensive care. It was in most cases a less traumatic way to transport them.

This is one of those transports.

Nice summer night, call volume down a little, and I was thinking that maybe I would have an easy night for a change. Then "she" called, a dispatcher who had the voice of a wounded African Gray, or maybe it was just the sheer repetition of her screeching, squawking voice creating that image and unpleasant association.

"Alpha 777, you have one in the emergency department of Boswell*, heading to William Randolph Hospital*." For clarification, William Randolph Hospital is a geriatric mental health facility located in an industrial suburb of the city of Detwah*, near the main airport servicing the greater Detwah metropolitan area. The importance of the facility's location will become clearer. On this particularly wonderful, warm Midwestern evening, the company paired me with a young, gung-ho basic EMT. My regular partner had taken the day off, and this young man decided to pick up an extra shift.

In addition to the newbie who had joined me, I was precepting a third rider. Many responders despised having student riders along on their shifts, an attitude that has always puzzled me. At some point in their EMS careers, those who now rejected teaching newbies had been part of the process, and *they* were the dreaded third rider. Riding third gave new EMTs hands-on experience under the guidance of an experienced EMT without the pressure of patient responsibility.

As part of their educational requirements, each brand-spanking-new EMT must log specified hours by riding with an experienced crew. Ride-time allows EMTs to gain valuable knowledge that not only helps them through the class but can also guide them toward a different career path. It is better to find out EMS is not the job for you under safe circumstances than when you are suddenly responsible for someone's life.

My newly assigned partner du jour and third rider were not familiar with my style of handling psychiatric transports. The most effective way to deal with these special-needs patients is by treating the psychiatric patient with the same respect offered to any medical patient and keeping their particular needs in mind for the safety of the patient and crew. Sometimes that respect came within seconds, simply by acknowledging the patient as an individual.

Making eye contact, introducing my partner and myself, and informing the patient about what would happen from the moment of our first contact until the patient arrived in the care of the receiving facility, showed respect. If appropriate, and if the transporting facility allowed a patient to ride unrestrained, sometimes I gave the patient a choice. Asking, "Would you like to ride (on the gurney) or walk to the ambulance" gave a patient some control over his situation and formed a bond of trust.

My regular partner was well aware of my philosophy regarding mental health patients and could play along with me in almost any situation. He understood my established patient handling patterns and nonverbal cues. We regularly visited facilities where the staff knew of our methods and gladly followed our lead, which we established through the carefully chosen words used during verbal reports.

These methods and communications often minimized the need for more restrictive and physical interventions, such as applying wrist and ankle restraints on patients. Because my regular partner had abandoned me for the day, I realized as we arrived at our dispatched location that it might be in my best interest to minimize interaction between the patient and my untrained and unaware fellow responders.

Boswell Hospital was a busy urban facility that did a good job of taking care of the residents living in their city. Our patient, Mr. Hersler[*], had waited patiently for our arrival. The unit nurse, after an exchange of pleasantries, conveyed to me that Mr. Hersler was going to be an issue. Hersler had to this point refused to communicate with staff, stating that he was *Captain* Hersler, and refused to talk to civilians regarding his involvement in the war. The nurse wished me well, adding that the patient had clothing in a bag under his cot but refused to get dressed.

I looked at the new EMT and the student rider, whose uniform was neatly pressed and looking very professional. The student was trying his best to look like a member of the crew with a stethoscope looped around his neck, and brand new navy blue pants and white shirt expertly pressed and unmarred by experience. My plan of action was to persuade Mr. Hersler to allow transport to a facility that would care for him and address his issues. As I approached Mr. Hersler, I made a quick self-check to see that my uniform took on at least a semblance of authority, and in a firm voice addressed the patient.

"Are you Hersler?"

"Yes."

At this point, I turned to tell "the men" that we would not need the transport cot and instructed them to wait by the transport vehicle. Mr. Hersler was peeking out from under the sheet and blankets that covered him from his toes to the bridge of his nose; he asked me who I was and what did I want.

"Captain Hersler, my name is Colonel Tompos. I am the commander of the 23rd bomber squadron, and your presence is required at headquarters for a briefing. We have little time to spare, and I insist that you ready yourself for transport."

At that moment, Mr. Hersler leaped from the cot in all his naked glory and offered me a proper salute, at which point the nurse behind the counter was making every effort to keep from laughing aloud. I often wondered whom the nurse found more amusing: Mr. Hersler, or me.

"Hersler, we do not have time for small talk. I order you to dress quickly so we can begin this journey. I also order you not to speak to the officers that have accompanied me since their security clearances are in question, is that understood?"

"Yes, *sir.*"

Mr. Hersler dressed quickly and accompanied me to the nurses' station to collect his "orders." Envelope in hand, Mr. Hersler and I stopped so that I could instruct him further.

"Captain Hersler, this trip will not take long, and I again stress avoiding conversation with the men accompanying me. Headquarters is near the airport, and when we are close you will notice aircraft (remember my earlier advisement that the receiving facility was near the airport). Upon arrival at the facility, the sergeant of arms will escort you to the meeting. Is that understood?"

"Yes, sir."

"They will question you and determine a plan of action."

The walk to the ambulance with a dressed Captain Hersler, and the drive to the hospital, was completely uneventful except for the wonderings of a puzzled student rider who did not understand why a patient would converse openly with me but completely ignore the student. A very short time later, we arrived safely at our destination.

At William Randolph Hospital, as part of established policy, security escorted EMS staff and ambulatory patients to their destination on the second floor. We knew from experience that the person who handled security most of the time was a very large, well-built man with very little tolerance for small talk. Ex-military, this man's habit was to speak only the last name of the patient and then instruct the patient and EMS staff to come with him.

Upon entering the facility with Mr. Hersler, my anticipated friend from security appeared wearing an expectedly well-pressed uniform, standing erect, large in stature, with eyes looking straight forward. He addressed my patient.

"You Hersler?"

"Yes, sir."

"Come with me!"

"Yes, sir."

Captain Hersler turned and saluted me. I know that somewhere in his mind, he lived in a bygone time and place. My job had been to get him to the appropriate level of care with a minimum of intervention: mission accomplished. I sharply returned the salute and dismissed my men. After returning to our ambulance, I took the time to explain what I had done and why. I wanted my protégés to understand that my actions and rationale were a means to an end, a method to deliver the patient to the help he needed without additional mental or physical stress.

I think Captain Hersler would have agreed.

~ ~ ~

Rising attention to alternative medicine, comprehensive care, naturopathic practice, and nutrition, as related to prevention and healing, has become a major focus in modern health care. Internet research merges with Granny's Home Remedies and Elixirs, while patients take control of their health maintenance. It can be a good thing or a bad thing. Convincing anyone that their knowledge may smack of pseudoscience or lack professional and scientific backing does little to sway those who "know what they know." Here are a few bits of wisdom and insanity, sometimes related to medicine by a very thin thread, collected from an assortment of medical and emergency service professionals (and those who love them). Bon Appétit.

Myths, Medicine, and Mocking

Sarah M. has been working in an ER since high school, so it comes as no surprise that she is now walking the educational path toward becoming an emergency physician. Flying between medical school and home is tiresome, but provides many opportunities to meet unique people. On one such trip, Sarah was talking to a woman who, when hearing Sarah was a medical student, launched into her view of all things medicine.

Perhaps the intent was for Sarah to benefit from years of the woman's accumulated pearls of wisdom. Perhaps the woman was encouraging Sarah to keep abreast of effective treatments that medical school may overlook. The woman had strong feelings about home remedies as alternative medicine.

Sarah reports in all earnestness, "I met an elderly lady at the airport who told me that she'd quit seeing her doctor because he didn't know how a hot mustard menthol rub on the chest helped her cough!" Unabashedly unthinkable! I am quite sure Sarah will bring that treatment to her professors and fellow students the moment she returns to school.

Or not.

~ ~ ~

As a cop, Tim H. worked the streets since before I was in kindergarten, encountering all kinds of explanations for behaviors and the cognitive reasoning behind them. These days, Tim is working paramilitary emergency services and runs the disaster response show for his state when airplanes fall out of the sky. When Tim shares memories or theories developed from his years on the road, I listen intently. He claims studies prove "Sex cures a headache. Really!"

Giving Tim the benefit of the doubt, I did a little research. Most of the studies I found were correlational for sex-related headaches and *gender*. Maybe Tim just misread the study.

~ ~ ~

Candida D. is a friend from back in high school. She is an intelligent, highly educated professional who gets as big a chuckle as I do from things that step outside of fact-based, empirical, reproducible, scientific evidence. Candida's mother "claimed that rubbing a raw potato on warts would eliminate them," which falls under the category of homebrews and wives' tales. However, giving me something that may have personal applications, Candida told me that her mother also "cut my brother's hair on the full moon. [She] claimed it grew back thicker."

I like that last one, and since it is a full moon, I may have to get a trim. Do not judge. At some time or another, almost all of us believe what we like, and discard the rest, no?

~ ~ ~

B.C. is a very dear friend who wore a uniform as a street cop before becoming a detective. It may be a stretch to see this situation as medical, but play along with me for a moment. Many years ago, B.C. stopped a woman for speeding, and the woman's excuse for exceeding the posted speed limit was a weak bladder. She was racing to get to the nearest bathroom. As a mid-century modern myself, with a bladder capacity of 125 ml, I can empathize.

B.C. was, unfortunately, not buying the excuse (he had heard them all) until the woman demonstrated her sincerity. B.C. sat in his car running the woman's identification through LEIN and NCIC while the speeder stood on the side of the road next to her car. As BC glanced into his rearview mirror, he saw the woman's khaki pants darken as she relieved herself. B.C. composed himself (until he drove away), and gave the woman back her identification. She did not get the ticket.

Anyone who has ever worked in a teaching facility will tell you to stay away from the ER whenever possible, but especially in July. May the Heavens, Angels, and all manner of good luck charms, the benefit of Karma, and any human-supporting extraterrestrials shine down upon you with mercy if you need to visit the ER on any *first* day of July. July 1st is the day the new residents, finally legally referring to themselves as "doctor" while wearing brand new standard-issue long white coats, descend upon us.

These new doctors will work 3-4 years in their residency to become board-certified emergency physicians, and the first day of practice is usually hazardous. Have no fear; the veteran ER nurse is watching over everything the new MD (or DO) is doing and ordering. If your nurse is out of sight, know that your ER Tech (often a paramedic with extremely advanced skills) has one eye on the resident at all times.

Please understand that I love my residents. I have raised many from pups and still have contact with them. Learning curves exist in all manner of professions, but Emergency Medicine has no room for error. We have to trust one another in the ER, as in EMS, and that trust and level of non-verbal communication can make a huge difference in patient care and outcomes. So bear with us in July, as we take baby steps to form useful communications and methods of working with one another, especially when some residents announce to staff, "I am the doctor, you are the nurse. Remember that."

Oh, we remember it. We remember it when newbie docs order enough medication to kill an elephant. If they respect us, we will not only respect them, we will take good care of them. We will mother them, feed them, watch over them, and teach them all of the tricks we learned over our many years working trauma centers. If the brand new former short coat comes in with an attitude, life could be hard; remember Karma, and that one reaps what one sows. For patients and families partaking of this combination plate of myth and mocking in medicine, please remember that I warned you.

~ ~ ~

The next warning related to the July 1 phenomenon involves mocking only those who have brought bad Karma upon themselves. A good number of brand-spanking-new residents were telling patients they were doctors all during their four years of medical school, but their short coats gave them away. Any ER staff member who overheard the inaccurate introductions ("Hi, I'm Doctor Smith") was quick to warn the first imprecise utterance with a raised eyebrow, the second time with an "excuse me?" and the third with a correction in front of the patient:

"Mrs. Widmayer, this is Jane Smith. She is a medical student who will be seeing you today if that is all right with you. Our supervising physician will oversee your care, and Jane will report to Dr. Don. Is that right, Jane? By the way, Mrs. Widmayer, you can tell the medical *students* from the resident *doctors* by their short white coats. Do you see Jane's short white coat, Mrs. Widmayer? That is how you know the difference."

A very dear friend of mine (Rick L.) suffered the wrath of ER nurses, some baring fangs, during his ER physician residency rotation. Unlike many new residents, as a previously practicing paramedic, Rick was experienced with emergency medicine, unlike those who come in with book knowledge and no experience. I was sorry Rick was not able to match with my hospital because I would have protected him. Some nurses are not so nice to medical students and residents.

Matter of fact, some nurses are not so nice to nurse newbies, as they continue to eat their young. Sadly, the practice lives through the negativity of some very old and cantankerous nurses, and I am just not referring only to the treatment of new graduate nurses. Nurses who have become the ranking big-fish in a small pond feel threatened by anyone coming in from another place. We are working on changing that practice, but change happens slowly. To quote Rodney King's famous declaration in 1992, "People, I just want to say can we all get along? Can we stop making it... horrible... It is just not right... it is not going to change anything."

Mode: Rant/off.

~ ~ ~

Mary tells of a personal encounter with an officer, which reinforces the myth that police officers avoid getting their highly polished boots soiled (who can blame them?). Mary had been speeding along above the posted limit, so when the officer activated his lights and siren, Mary pulled over and thought quickly about how to evade a deserved ticket. Opening her car door and leaning out as the officer approached (calculated risk in Detroit), Mary put her hand over her mouth.

"Officer, *gag* I'm sorry, *gag* I know I was speeding, *gag* but I've been throwing up all night, and I'm going to the ER. Stand back, *gag* I don't want to puke on your shoes." Mary was convincing, swaying, and moaning for effect, as she saw the officer's boots slowly retreat. She heard him tell her to shut her door and continue to the hospital.

The officer wanted assurance that Mary was sincere, so he followed behind her. Sure enough, Mary pulled into the ER parking lot, so the officer returned to the streets. Had the officer paused for a moment, he would have seen Mary walking toward the ER doors wearing scrubs and a hospital badge. Mary was indeed going to the ER, but she was an employee speeding along because she was late for work.

~ ~ ~

Suzanne is a wonderful RN who, for reasons that escape my understanding, wants to deliver babies for a living. In EMS, left lateral recumbent was my favorite position for laboring women (lying on their left sides to keep from delivering). My accompanying instruction for the driver was, "Go fast." Because Suzanne deals with a lot of folklore that accompanies pregnancy, she reminded me of the old (false) advice for pregnant women not to put their arms over their heads, lest the cord wrap around the baby's neck (a nuchal cord). Babies are mostly unaffected by mom's movements during pregnancy, although walking up to pregnant women and shaking their belly with both hands may be a little irritating to the incubating babe and the mom.

My daughter, Missy has photographic proof of that last statement. During an ultrasound, as the technician rolled her wand disturbingly over Andrew's domain (Missy's belly), the boy put both hands over his eyes as if to say, "Seriously?" Scrutiny of the 4-D photograph shows the depth of Andrew's feelings, as one fist displays an extended middle finger.

Mocking? Indeed.

~ ~ ~

This myth, with a medical basis in fact (which is where many myths begin) involves garlic. Suzanne shares patient wisdom about placing a clove of peeled garlic in the ear to combat infections. The active ingredient used in prepared garlic oils contains allicin, purported as an antibiotic and antifungal, but using a regular clove of garlic can be dangerous. Some folks have foolishly tried to mash and chop several cloves of garlic and then, mixing the mash with water, shoot the concoction into their ears with a syringe.

I recall Mama advising not to put anything larger than my elbow in my ear (or maybe that was a commercial for Q-Tips). I have also heard those who tried to use several cloves of remedial garlic, thinking if one is good six is better, that it is an incredibly painful experience. Crossing chef shows with healing can get a little muddled, and going to the ER to have bits of garlic removed from one's ear(s) is downright embarrassing. Nonetheless, some folks swear by the healing powers of garlic. I support naturopathy and homeopathy, but this practice can go very, very wrong.

~ ~ ~

Suzanne mentions another abuse of garlic, something that she, as a practicing registered nurse, has encountered: placing garlic in the vagina for a yeast infection. I am tying my fingers in a knot right now to resist writing down all the mental places that particular gem allows my mind to go. Feel free to put this book down and think about it for a few minutes. I will be here when you get back.

(I pause briefly. I get up and stretch. I take a drink of sugar-free, raspberry-flavored iced green tea. I pet Izzy, my cat. I throw a toy mouse expecting Izzy to retrieve it and play fetch; he does not. I consider making popcorn but decide that breaking another tooth on a popcorn kernel is too expensive.)

More Confessions of a Trauma Junkie

I cannot do it; I cannot let this one go. For a moment, and we are viewing this completely from a clinical perspective, and quite professionally, imagine that a female patient literally inserts a clove of garlic into her vagina and goes to bed. If she is at all like the ear people, she may peel and insert several (if one is good, six is better, remember?).

In the morning, she realizes she cannot locate the garlic clove(s) either in her bed or in her Va-Jay-Jay. Thinking that gravity will help, she goes about her business, probably more comfortable since the antimicrobial properties of the garlic worked their magic (or she did not have a yeast infection).

The busy girl that she is, Sally Sunshine* forgets about her misplaced garlic remedy. A few days later, a very distinctive and unpleasant odor that she cannot identify permeates Sally's home. She checks the garbage disposal, looks under the sinks in the kitchen and bathroom, empties all the trash containers in the house, sprays Lysol with one hand and Febreeze with the other on everything, and lights scented candles. The noxious smell seems to follow her.

Sally finally realizes that she is the source of the odor, which gives a completely new meaning to the words "crotch rot" (my EMS and ER friends were *waiting* for that one). Sally drives to the ER and presents to the triage nurse with a complaint of "foreign object/vagina." The second nurse and attending physician see the chart and assume Sally has lost a tampon, which is a very common complaint. Because of the risk of TSS (Toxic Shock Syndrome), the professional folks take the complaint seriously and prepare for examination.

Sally is ushered into a private "girl" room containing a table with the lovely cold, metal stirrups all females have learned to loathe. Prepped by the nurse who now knows why Sally has come to a busy emergency room for a week-old complaint, Sally feels her heart thumping and face warming from embarrassment. The nurse holds her breath, exits the room, and tells the doctor through tears streaming down her face that the patient is ready for her pelvic exam.

On the instrument table that the nurse prepared for the examination, next to the sterile cup for the garlic, are ring forceps to retrieve the clove(s) and a mask for the doctor. The nurse will explain to Sally that garlic is toxic, so the doctor is wearing the mask, with a plastic face shield, to protect his eyes. If the doctor cannot visualize the garlic, he may have to send the patient for very expensive testing to locate the foreign objects, and the word unpleasant does not even begin to describe Sally's adventure.

Thus ends our foray into Imaginary Sally and the Va-Jay-Jay garlic—for now—but if I hear from anyone who has had this situation in his or her ER (or ambulance), there will be a sequel. I will not be able to help myself.

~ ~ ~

Kojak* reminisces about responding as a patrol officer many years ago to a certain motor vehicle accident. A female had rear-ended a car and was screaming at the owner of the car she'd hit. The woman claimed to have swallowed a tube of lipstick when the accident occurred and fully intended to sue the other driver not only for damages in the accident but also for the cost of the lipstick.

Through her screaming, the woman displayed more than adequate lung capacity, so the officers immediately ruled out any medical emergency involving problems with a foreign object in the airway. The woman continued her verbal diatribe, insisting that the other driver, a pleasant and calm man, had stopped short in front of her. Witnesses contradicted those claims, saying the man stopped at the light 10-15 seconds before the woman had hit him, so the accident was her fault.

The woman had been applying lipstick "while looking in the rearview mirror," according to Kojak. She failed to see the man stopped in front of her vehicle and "creamed him." Kojak issued a ticket for reckless driving as opposed to a simple failure to reduce speed to avoid based on her statement "about putting on the lipstick and subsequently swallowing it due to the crash." Kojak addresses the applicable medical mockery with the doctor's statement about the woman swallowing the tube of lipstick: "That too shall pass."

Kojak did not follow up on the disposition of the lipstick.

~ ~ ~

Earlier I mentioned that sometimes we are not sure whose reality is real. If someone is operating under a system of beliefs that differ from ours, are their spiritual visions a fantasy? Alternatively, are they perhaps so in touch with their belief systems that they completely understand and embrace things that we have only read about, seen on television, or heard anecdotally? Sometimes it is hard to tell, but professionally, we respond to standards, norms of culture, society, and the common practices between people regionally. If someone brings their practices, for which we have no understanding, and worse yet, treat with fear and loathing, outcomes are unpredictable. Ultimately, we emergency services folks stick with the medical, follow protocols, fear the worst, and hope for the best.

Possession is 9/10ths of the Psyche

After sitting safely and contentedly in one's living room watching television or a movie about the spooky side of life with friends and family, fears about the great unknowns of this world disappear when the light comes on. Sometimes you keep that light on for several nights in a row if the things witnessed were especially disturbing, but looking around confers some measure of reassurance. Either those things seen and heard were a product of Hollywood special effects, or they happened so far away from you that your fears are unrealistic and will eventually disappear. For some, those moments of fear are fun because they are not a shared reality. They do not exist.

In EMS, we have seen things that completely confound us. Some of our patients have experiences or visions that we do not share, nor do we understand them. When cultures merge, folks who bring practices with them that seem completely normal (to them) make the hairs on the back of our necks stand up. Hair-raising does not begin to describe what happened when Paramedic Jeff S. and I responded to a call in a migrant farm area outside city limits.

The dispatched complaint was "woman having a seizure," which can mean anything, so our only level of mental preparation was for a medical emergency involving a female. The dispatch information did not give an address, directing us to a field near two named cross streets. I began to develop an icky feeling in the pit of my stomach, sensing something was not right. Fearless Jeff was up for anything, but I was preparing myself mentally and emotionally for the unknown.

It was summertime, and migrant farmhands from all over the world inhabited the area for seasonal work. Summer nights were warm and especially humid. The word sticky comes to mind, and our polyester shirts and pants, great for appearances because they came out of the dryer looking pressed, clung to us unmercifully. We knew the area of the cross streets well because they approached the county line, and in that area there were only stars to light our way. No streetlights, no porch lights, no commercial buildings. Nothingness shrouded in darkness.

We arrived on the scene to find two police cars and a fire vehicle marking the entry point to the woods. The police informed us that our female patient had been performing animal sacrifice, probably a voodoo ritual, when she began having seizure-like activity that concerned those with her. Grateful to stay behind, I set up our equipment as Jeff accompanied the police, pulling our stretcher prepared with a long backboard and extra straps deeper into the woods. The dancing lights of the officer's flashlights were the last images I saw, and then I was alone.

I had always maintained a healthy fear of darkness, the night, and the supernatural. Jeff was looking forward to an adventure. I was wondering if we were about to usher demons into our Emergency Room on Wheels, blessings, and exorcisms at no extra charge. If demons followed the woman into our rig, would they follow us home? I mentally gathered an armor of appropriate scriptures, reciting them softly as I waited.

Jeff told me later that when he found the woman, she was thrashing about, foaming at the mouth, and uttering sounds best described as inhuman. The patient was growling and spitting, so (in a time before spit hoods), Jeff put a simple mask over her face to protect us, the firefighters, and the officers from any possible diseases transmitted through her saliva. Three police officers, four firefighters, and Jeff struggled to restrain the woman, who seemed unaware of her surroundings, and angry that the men were interfering with her ritual. She never spoke, although she responded to things verbalized to her with a deep and menacing growl.

When the men loaded our patient into the ambulance, she was not seizing. She continued to growl at Jeff, who laughed as she spat because she succeeded only in spitting back on her face inside the mask. The woman was not verbalizing in any discernible language and was acting inappropriately, so police requested that we take her to the hospital for medical evaluation.

The officers provided the necessary paperwork allowing us to take the woman against her will. When someone does not want to go to the hospital but appears medically unstable, we have a legal duty to transport them. If there is any question about the appropriateness of the transport, police can write a petition ordering hospital evaluation, absolving EMS of legal responsibility for transporting someone against their will.

Our struggle with the patient continued in the rear of the ambulance as six of us attempted to secure her for transport. The patient was strapped to a backboard and secured by a KED board. With the dexterity of a circus contortionist, she continued to pull one limb after another out of the secured straps. Jeff decided that both of us should attend to the patient in the back of the rig, and a volunteer firefighter drove our ambulance to the hospital.

The ride was eerie, but there was no movie to turn off, no escape into another room. The woman continued to growl and sneer at us. We battled to keep her secured (for her safety as well as ours) during the perceptual eternity of the 15-minute ride.

Her facial expressions reminded me of when I saw a bat dying in a closed jar, and I hoped that if she was devil-possessed, the demons would stay with her. I felt as though I were in the presence of one who had opened a portal to Hell, and each time she looked into my eyes, searing pain stabbed psyche, attempting to penetrate my soul. I could hear her laughter mock my spirituality as she challenged us. There was an inexplicable, threatening, dark presence.

I cannot honestly say if this was a demonic situation, but I will admit placing a mental white light of protection around myself. Sometimes the most powerful enemies are unseen, and we wonder if we are sufficiently prepared to battle them. I washed the rig out with extra Big Orange citrus-scented cleaner to banish the unwanted evil spirits and hoped for an uneventful completion of my 24-hour shift.

Moreover, I slept with the lights on.

~ ~ ~

Mental illness, illicit drugs, alcohol, chemical dependencies, sedentary lifestyles without ambition, and reasoning as solid as Swiss cheese can all contribute to convoluted perspectives on life. Along our professional journey in ES, we encounter folks approaching every challenge through a side door, for whatever reason, and often we cannot come to a meeting of the minds.

Mental Notes on Paper

Working ER triage is a challenging job reserved for the most experienced and discerning ER staff. Trying to sort between drama and trauma takes a trained eye and years of skill development. Most ERs will not let a staff member manage the front triage desk, no matter how many years they may have in other facilities, until they have been in that particular hospital at least six months. As the first warm body between the door and the docs, the person out front needs to know either the answer to every question or where to find it.

One type of patient is visually identifiable from a distance of 25 feet. Those who come in to admit themselves for psychiatric help or evaluation carry at least a week's worth of clothing, snacks, creature comforts (like cigarettes), and lots of reading material. The suitcase is often the maximum size allowed on aircraft and bursting at the seams.

If the ER is full, this patient creates challenges for the triage nurse, because if the patient utters the magic words, "I have suicidal ideations," they not only go immediately back to see the doc but also earn a staff member to sit with them for safety. When the problem is legitimate, we are happy to be of service. Folks abusing the complaint to bypass a full waiting room are another story.

ER Techs have the worst job in these situations. The techs are responsible for taking comprehensive inventories of the contents of the suitcases. Without a comprehensive belongings list, patients get to their rooms and suddenly realize their $150 sneakers, $6,000 Breitling watches, and multiple pieces of diamond jewelry are missing. One particular day some years ago, I remember a patient who topped the charts in audacity.

The very tiny woman could barely pull her wheeled suitcase up to the triage desk. She reported having suicidal ideations after a drug binge and wanted help getting off drugs. The patient knew that without the suicidal ideation complaint, social work would give her resource materials for rehabilitation centers and send her on her way. Saying she had suicidal ideations (words shared by those familiar with the system, as "ideations" was the only polysyllabic word in this patient's lexicon) guaranteed a psychiatric evaluation and hospital stay of at least 72 hours.

Triage Nurse: "Why are you here?"

Patient: "I have suicidal ideations."

Triage Nurse: "Do you have a plan?"

Patient: "I have a gun at home, and if you don't admit me I will blow my brains out" (women usually employ less violent means, but this is her story).

Triage Nurse: "OK; let's get you to a room, and the doctor will see you shortly."

Back in the patient care area, another nurse helped the patient out of her clothes and into a gown. As she put the belongings into a plastic see-through patient property bag, marked with the patient's name and medical record number, the nurse heard the tech standing outside the curtain say, "I need security here. Now!" Throwing the curtain back, the nurse saw the tech frozen in place with his hands up in the air as though someone said, "This is a stick-up."

The patient had prepared quite well for this trip. In addition to the normal creature comforts one might pack for a weeklong "hospital vacation," this patient brought an impressive stash of cocaine, marijuana, and several unidentifiable pills placed randomly into tiny, Ziploc bags. Security came and confiscated all of the drugs, saying the patient had enough illegal drugs to sell to the whole hospital and had stuffed an extra crack pipe inside her folded socks.

The tech and nurse signed the security envelope, relieved to have the stash out of their work area. Security officers contacted the local PD. No one in the ER heard what happened when, upon release, the patient asked for her missing valuables, but I am sure the staff directed her to the local police precinct.

I wonder if she ever called.

~ ~ ~

None of us, neither emergency services folks nor civilians, can avoid crises. At some point in life, everybody becomes involved in at least one crisis. Whether it happens to us or someone we love, situations that are clearly beyond normal circumstances and experience happen (also known as "Doo-doo Occurs"). Things that go bump in the night present images and sensory assaults that fill our psyche and our souls.

Some folks believe that we unconsciously choose these challenges to allow our spirits to evolve. Some think that we call these events to ourselves because of the thoughts we project into the universe. Others proffer that it is dumb luck, chance, or being in the wrong place at the wrong time. Whatever the explanation-defying rationale, the unexpected can send our logical minds reeling in a desperate search to understand tragedies we inevitably encounter.

We can become stuck. Like an old movie reel, images repeat in our minds without end, a continuous loop. We try to make sense of the situation, but some things defy logic. No matter how deftly we handle creative problem-solving personally and professionally, or how sharp our critical thinking skills, some things are beyond our intellectual or emotional capacity. How do we make sense of the senseless?

There is no logic to a mother becoming so stoned on drugs that she rolls over on her baby, suffocating him between couch cushions because mom "forgot" the baby was there. There is no answer to the wondering of why bad things happen to kind and loving people. No neat compartmentalization exists in which to file the pointless tragedies that happen every day. Emergency services folks responding to these tragedies often expect to work miracles, and when that does not happen, some of us take it very personally.

We come with lights flashing and sirens blaring to do the impossible. That is what drives us. I have an inner child who thinks that hopeless situations are simply a challenge to life's rules.

If we do the right thing in the right way at the right time with the right intent, we increase the chances of success. That illusion of control supports the belief that nothing happens by chance. We want to influence random events, affecting outcomes to create happy endings. Unfortunately, endings are not always happy or successful.

We see the types of things that make for entertaining television and movies and walk away unaffected. Using our skills and training is invigorating and rewarding. Most of us, most of the time, come through unscathed, and even if we are affected, we survive by ourselves or with support systems.

I do not want to give the impression that all of us are freaking out all of the time; quite the opposite is true. Becoming emotionally stuck is the exception rather than the rule. The problem is that we do not know with certainty, beyond predictive probability, what will affect whom or in what way.

One post-crisis intervention tool involves taking a bad incident and finding something positive about it, giving value to the experience. A mother loses a child to suicide because of Internet bullying and brings folks together to change legislation. An emergency services worker sees his coworkers succumbing to the emotional aftereffects of trauma and introduces an organizational crisis response plan. With crisis intervention, a firefighter who responds to a house fire killing three of four inhabitants discovers a way to reframe the mental picture, gaining the perspective that he did not lose three people, he *saved* one!

Most of us act positively in response to moments when the pendulum swings so widely out of balance that we are sure the earth is about to topple. Recognizing those moments and reframing the picture to find the glass-half-full side of the equation keeps our sanity intact. Finding even the smallest success in what others term disaster allows us to refuel our tanks, stay healthy, grow stronger, and come back to work another day.

Mental note on paper: look for the good, tolerate and educate those who cannot find it, and focus on how to make things better.

Amen.

~ ~ ~

One of my biggest pet peeves in the ER relates to staff treating patients seeking emotional help as though they were born of a lesser God. Sometimes there exists a very fine and almost imperceptible line between reality and imagination, between sanity and the mental darkness that envelops people after tragedy marks their lives. It is completely normal to be depressed after significant loss, and asking for help. Under those circumstances, is not a sign of weakness, but of strength.

The affected person can sink into a foreign and uncomfortable place, with nothing to look forward to but plunging even deeper. Places of helplessness and hopelessness do not exist only for "other people." Any one of us might come upon just the right circumstances at some point in our lives and become that "psych" patient. Maybe we already have.

I was dealing with a young woman whose whole world began to disintegrate before her eyes after discovering that her husband had been unfaithful. She did not know how to take the next breath, much less figure out what to do in a situation she had never anticipated. Her worldview, her future, and most of how she remembered her relationship's past suddenly changed.

The woman thought she was surely damaged or inferior, or it would never have happened. She had nowhere to turn, considered ending her life, but realized that a permanent answer to a temporary problem was not logical. Her heart longed for relief that would not come, and she did not know if the pain would ever end. She felt as though she were breathing a fire that seared her lungs but would not kill her. She wanted to stop hurting so intensely.

The woman registered with ER triage as having severe depression and, when asked if she had ever considered suicide, said, "I just want to go to sleep and not wake up." That declaration did not mean she was suicidal, but standard precautions assured her safety until the doctor or social worker could make a professional determination. The woman's clothing, bagged and secured, moved to the nurse's station, and the patient donned a dark green gown, designating her as a psychiatric patient. The color-coding system lets staff know that anyone in a green gown merits watchful eyes.

The tech assigned to the ER Behavioral Health holding area that day loved working with psych patients. It was easy: bag the clothes, take vital signs once a shift, walk patients to the bathroom as needed, and give them food. Unlike the rest of the ER, after completing those minor tasks for a maximum of six patients, the tech was to "sit," which meant sitting in view of his patients to ensure none absconded.

Hospitals hire people called sitters who sit, watch the patients, and advise if a psych patient tries to flee. The sitters do not take vital signs or assist the nurse or patient in any way. They sit, usually reading magazines or doing their homework, though some are diligent about keeping an eye on the patients. Some sitters take their jobs literally, and if a patient tries to run out the doors, the sitter will yell the nurse's name from their chair, never getting up at all, even if the nurse is nowhere in sight. They sit.

My depressed patient, who was already having serious issues with self-esteem following the discovery of her husband's philandering, took a particular dislike to the tech assigned to her. I thought perhaps it was a personality issue, but when the patient became suddenly tearful after an encounter with the young man, I asked her what had happened. She told me that he had been negative and verbally abusive to her since she came into the ER.

He was rude, condescending, and referred to her as "L2K" (a legal designation for psychiatric hold patients) instead of by her name. She finally asked what had she had done to make him so angry and inconsiderate. He said nothing, so she insisted upon an answer, asking, "Why are you treating me like this?"

The tech said, "Because I can."

When she told me her story, I apologized for her mistreatment and had the tech removed from the area until the physician could talk with the patient. While another nurse covered for me, I took a short dinner break and used the time to ask other nurses if they had ever had this type of experience. Each had a story about that tech's bad attitudes, outbursts of anger, insubordination, extended breaks, and inappropriate conversations.

When I got back to my work area, the woman was gone. She had run out of the building, and the sitter who was with her did not get up to stop her. The sitter said she'd called for the nurse, but by the time the nurse returned from the locked med-room, where the nurse could not have heard anyone calling her name, the patient was "OTD" (out the door).

We called the police and reported the woman's escape, the situation, and wrote the incident up for the supervisors. The male tech never again worked with the psych patients (thankfully), but it was too late for this young woman in her time of need, a woman who trusted medical professionals to act professionally.

I believe in Karma. I wonder if the woman ever found peace. I wonder if the emotionally abusive tech received some appropriate judgment (besides losing his job). I wonder if all of those who deal so impatiently and harshly with folks who are in pain will someday know what it feels like on the other side of the dark green gown.

~ ~ ~

Sometimes Karma is immediate. Again assigned to the Behavioral Health section of the ER, I worked with a female tech who was very strict about following rules. This tech took pride in her job and felt she was the leader of the unit. The nurse was simply there to do paperwork and hand out shots and pills. Because I did not work the "psych hold" section that often, I appreciated the tech's experience.

During the change of shift report, the off-going staff nurse delivered a caveat about one of the developmentally delayed patients in my care. The patient became violent if he heard the word "No." I relayed the information to my tech and thought no more about it. Generally, the tech was completely competent and very personable, but on this day failed to respect the wisdom behind the off-going nurse's warning. When the patient asked the tech for more juice, she declared that he had already had more than enough, and sternly told the young man, *"NO!"*

The impressive finger wound from the boy clamping down with very healthy teeth onto the tech's finger required a good cleaning, some steri-strips, and a tetanus shot. Karma.

~ ~ ~

Have you ever thought about how much influence we have (or do not have) over aging and the physiological changes that occur over time? For example, if aging speeds up with certain biological processes (like stress or disease), then we should be able to manipulate slowing the aging process. Progeria, the aging disease, baffles us, but finding the etiology (cause) might mean finding a cure. Slowing the rapid aging process of that disease could conceivably work to slow the detrimental cellular destruction of aging in otherwise healthy people, and perhaps affect the processes of other diseases.

Cells have a memory and a shelf life, and we know we can speed aging by doing bad things to our bodies (sun worshiping, smoking, eating too much of the wrong things, sedentary lifestyles). What if we do what our bodies need (however that is determined) to keep the cells healthier? I know of folks who smoked and drank and lived to the ripe old age of 103, but I wonder if the bad habits were protective factors, or if the folks had a genetic predisposition to live even longer had they not indulged.

Then there is perception and the old physics rules regarding energy before matter. We think first, act second. Can we learn to take action, to influence our physiology during that undefined space between thoughts, to someday, somehow accomplish improving ourselves on a cellular level?

We know that chronic stress has dynamic pathological effects on the body, quantifiable physiological responses, and measurable permanent changes to the brain (as with severe traumatic stress and alcoholism). Why not learn to have a reversing biopsychosocial self-effect? Psychologists delved deeply into our psyche and actions in discovering and defining learned behavior. If we can learn, why not *un*learn (which is to say learn another way, or replace previous dysfunctional learning with positive perception)?

My big grudge with nursing eons ago during nursing school was the definition of nursing given by preceptors: "responding to the biopsychosocial effects of injury and illness." We did not spend much time proactively promoting health, wellness, and positivity. In emergency medicine, we lacked the opportunity to address more than immediate needs amid crises.

Must we follow pathology instead of an anti-pathology, proactive, health-seeking path that may affect our body's responses to illness, injury, or stress assaults in a less harmful way? Can we self-inoculate with positive perceptions? Can we create or encourage attitudes that are more buoyant, more resistant to the assaults, and more resilient when experiencing those challenges?

Many years ago, I read a book called *SuperImmunity: Master Your Emotions and Improve Your Health* by Paul Pearsall, Ph.D. Dr. Pearsall suggested that our bodies experience little skirmishes (colds, flu) waged in preparation for major battles (big gun diseases). We do physiological tabletop exercises, in essence training to fight larger threats should they come along. It made sense, and I began to look at things from that perspective.

I think we have the internal knowledge now, though we may not use it, or even be aware of it, to affect healing. Moreover, I believe that at some point we may come up with the medical answers (which most people believe instead of that "soft science" psychology stuff), allowing ourselves to believe in the power we possess over our biopsychosocial selves. Perception is everything, and the glass-half-full folks have a winning advantage.

Go ahead and call me a Pollyanna if your glass is half-empty. Research is on the side of the power of positivity. How cool is that?

POSTMORTEM

I wrote this book's first edition while in graduate school studying psychology, with a specialization in crisis management and response. The courses were very telling, answering many questions formed in childhood by a curious mind studying abnormal psychology from a very early age. Unfortunately, from personal experience I understand gaslighting, emotional and physical abuse, and the joys of being married to a sociopathic narcissist. Fortunately, I learned not to marry men anymore to save them, to deal with them as their nurse. I also learned none of us are exempt from PTSD from occupational or personal exposure.

My professional experience includes working with the mentally ill in locked units, in prison, and addiction medicine, detox, and rehab. Each was rewarding as my empathy grew outside my protective cocoon. A white light, a more developed trauma armor, enveloped me.

I decided when I had given enough, and learned not to let the patients take more than I wanted to give. Coworkers and management were often far more trouble and stress-inducing than patients. Anxiety increases with unmet expectations, so keeping hopes realistic went a long way toward being an effective and helpful nurse who did not lose her soul.

The addiction med folks held my heart. Watching their strides and movement toward sober living, their small realizations that led to major changes in their lives, their ability to get back up again, and again, and again renewed my belief in hope. Some of my coworkers talked about patients rolling through a "revolving door," failing to see that addiction changes the hard-wiring of the brain, and folks have to learn to live and work with an entirely new set of legos to build their lives. Some of them could not break the cycle, with heartbreaking outcomes. Some of them enjoyed great success, one day at a time.

There was one young man in particular who captured my heart, hope and continued prayers. He was incredibly intelligent, dealt with physical challenges, and had a very pronounced stutter. Most of the staff became impatient and finished his sentences instead of giving him time to complete his thoughts at his own pace. I gained an understanding as to how easily he might have stumbled into substance abuse as a coping mechanism.

One day he wrote a complaint about a staff member who brought with her from home personal problems and a bad attitude. The patient said he was treated poorly and disrespected. When he talked to me about his complaint, I listened, did not complete his thoughts for him, and he thanked me for being so professional. He looked at me and said, "they see this," pointing to his body, "but they don't know what's up here," tapping his forehead.

The day I prepared his discharge papers, knowing/hoping I would not see him again, I went to the cafeteria after my shift to find him and say goodbye. He smiled and cocked his head to the side when he saw me. I said I wanted to wish him well and offered my hand. He said, "No, I want a hug," clear as a bell, no stutter. I bent over his wheelchair, gave him a grandmotherly hug, and said, "Make good decisions."

Another patient was an older gentleman with mild dementia who had a rough start to his detoxification and rehab. As I began morning rounds, this gentleman was one of the few up and about. He told me about dreaming of a good southern home-cooked meal, that it was the first pleasant dream he had since starting rehab. He added, softly, as he looked at his shoes, "I wouldn't have gotten through except for a good doctor and good nurse. My gratitude and blessings are all I have to give." I thanked him, understanding that he truly gave me everything he had.

In retrospect, I have learned about being able to deliver care without jumping off an ambulance or running around an emergency room. Some ask, "You used to be a paramedic? Or, when were you a nurse?" As a retired paramedic and trauma nurse, changing where and how I practice involved learning to embrace lowered expectations and judgment.

Prison nursing was a huge part of that lesson as I saw men who had already been judged and lived with daily enforcement. They needed a safe place to go, where their crimes were not part of medical evaluation or treatment unless it affected my safety. Psychiatric and addictions nursing added to the knowledge that everyone has a story, and sometimes the only difference is a matter of uniform and keys. Far too often there is a fine line between "us" and "them." As professionals and humans we need to be careful not to trip over that line. Karma.

Part III | Both Sides of the Gurney

I must warn you that the first story in this section is about experiencing both sides of the gurney as an emergency services worker losing a parent, and the third story about losing a beloved pet. If you choose to skim over them, I understand completely. The section in the middle, however, is much lighter to give readers and this writer a break.

Switching gears from medical professionals to family members ideally happens with some notice and preparation. Sometimes those luxuries of forewarning and preparation bypass us at warp speed, and we do not know what has hit us. The only thing we know with any certainty is that this type of blow can be, emotionally, nearly fatal. Unlike movies where loved ones surround you, and new situations fall delicately, in real life, when the bomb drops, you are never prepared and often alone.

Stepping through Alice's Mirror

"This is Sandy* with Deckerville Ambulance. I am with your mom at her house, and she is not up to talking right now. She wanted me to call you, and I'm very sorry to tell you this, but your father has passed away."

I had taken the call in my home office, and after putting the phone back in the cradle, I walked in circles around the center of the small room, trying to figure out what to do. No one wants to hear on the telephone that his or her parent has died. I know Sandy did not want to be the one delivering that pronouncement.

As a medic, I did not have to make those types of calls. As a nurse, I was usually with a doctor when a patient's family received bad news. As difficult as the medic or nurses' job is in those situations, they trump being the daughter thrown into the deep end of the pool without knowing how to swim.

Attempting to find the safety of intellectualizing, a coping skill that had always served me well professionally, I tried to think logically, but could not. Still walking in circles, I felt a gasp come from somewhere deep inside that reminded me that I was not breathing. I think I heard myself say the word "no" several times, and it was in the voice of the child who was not prepared to let go of the dad she had not known long enough.

My Dad came into my life when I was nine years old. I was not quite sure how to handle the new arrangement since my only father figures were television actors, but a popular commercial cleverly answered the "But what do I call him?" question. I loved Tootsie Pops, and those who were around in the 1960s may remember the commercial, "Pop, Pop, Tootsie Pop... Daaaad."

The day my mom married my dad, I presented him with Tootsie Pops, said the line from the commercial, and never had to deal with the clumsiness surrounding a new stepparent's name again. As the only dad I ever really knew, he was not a stepparent at all. He was my Dad.

Mom and Dad left for their honeymoon but cut their trip short to come back for David and me. I cannot imagine a new groom coming back for the new kids (we were the only children my dad would ever have), but Dad embraced his new family immediately and fully. Mom liked to say she had a lousy husband, but her kids had a great father. We always came first in Dad's life.

The present reality was harsh, and there was no time for denial. The state police and the coroner were waiting in the driveway of my parents' home until I arrived because I was the keeper of all things medical. Dad was in the coroner's van.

Although every ounce of energy drained out of me, I knew my mom was waiting. I had to clear my head. Wading laboriously through the deep end of the emotional pool, still gasping for air, I picked up the phone to call my boss.

"Jan[*], I won't be at work tomorrow. My dad just died, and I am going up north to take care of things." Having worked crisis management, EMS, and ER for so many years, I knew the first thing folks say upon hearing of personal loss is, "I'm sorry." Waiting to hear those words before I hung up, I was surprised to hear, "Oh, I suppose this means I have to find someone to cover for you."

Thanks, Jan.

It felt like a rubber band snapped in the middle of my brain. ER nurses in our busy Detroit hospital normally had to find someone to take their shifts if they wanted time off, but this was different. Sorry Jan, but my dad failed to give adequate notice before dying, so I guess you'll have to find someone to take my shifts. It sucks to be you!

The mental detour gave me enough energy to throw some clothes into a duffel bag. Of course, I chose the red bag labeled "EMS," still trying to maintain professional distance. The nurse paramedic could handle this. Mike Dudley's little girl could not. Driving 90 miles north took forever as I raced toward the place I never wanted to reach.

The trip up the lakeshore wound through Port Huron, Lexington, and Port Sanilac. It was normally a beautiful and peaceful drive. Traveling down Lakeshore Drive had always meant taking deep breaths in and blowing all of my worries out toward the horizon of Lake Huron, usually settling them on a freighter off in the distance.

I had driven down that road countless times, working as a medic, sometimes on the wrong side of the road if we were "coding" to an emergency call, and John (an EMTS and police officer) was driving. John loved to say that if he drove on the right side of the road, no one would move to the side. If he drove on the wrong side of the road, they parted like the red seas. He was right.

This time I drove alone. There was no ambulance, no partner, no one to talk to, and no way to silence my brain. When responding to calls on the lakeshore, I often wondered what people thought about when they were waiting for the ambulance. Time must have stood still as they waited in the cold after an accident or stood helplessly next to the water's edge, not knowing if anyone would arrive in time to pull their child from the murky waters. Hundreds of calls over the years, and I saw so many of them reappear in my mind as I drove the lakeshore this time, this surreal time.

Turn left off the lakeshore, travel seven miles. There was Mom and Dad's house, a beautiful stone house set back from the others. Many years before, a farmer took his horse and buggy those seven miles every day to Lake Huron and pulled stones from the water's edge, then brought them back to form another row on the exterior of his house. On this day, there was a police car, coroner's vehicle, and the three men who operated those vehicles standing in the driveway.

I walked up to them with my red EMS bag over my shoulder, trying to look somewhat composed, and introduced myself. The officer opened a notebook, the small pocket-sized spiral-bound standard police issue that I used in EMS, and asked about my dad's medical history. "Sixtry-five-year-old male, history of congested cardiomyopathy, ejection fraction of 15%, medically managed with several cardiac medications…"

I remember words coming out my mouth like a report I would give about any patient I might deliver to the local ER. The words rang hollow. I looked into the eyes of the officers for some recognition that we were on the same team, but I was not in uniform, and they didn't know me. I was an outsider.

Maybe I had hoped to pull some strength and support from my brothers in blue. EMS in our small town was part of the police station, so we were on the same team. I hoped somehow they would recognize that connection, and share some support to keep me upright. This day I was just some woman they had been waiting for before they could call back in service, have lunch, or go home. I cannot remember what time of day it was, only that it was daylight.

I was on the other side of the mirror.

I was the daughter, not the medic or nurse. I was just another family member outside of the room of uniforms, outside of that inner sanctum, where I had felt safe and protected. My voice had been echoing in my head, but it did not match what I was thinking or saying. At one point, I was not even sure if I was talking aloud, watching for a reaction from the others to indicate whether I was thinking or speaking.

The two sides of the mirror blurred, and I stood with an arm on each side, hoping my façade held long enough to give the three men all the information they needed. I thought I was completely professional, but that illusion broke into piercing slivers of glass, bringing droplets of blood nearer to the surface of my psyche. The coroner, who was just a local funeral director granted extra titles in a small town, abruptly ended my report with his diagnosis.

"So he died of CHF."

I felt my face flush. I objected; my dad did not have CHF. My dad never had CHF (congestive heart failure). He had an arrhythmia that made him a candidate for sudden death from his heart beating in a non-life-supporting, wacky way. That is how many folks die from heart problems. Therefore, the logical choice was sudden cardiac arrest, not congestive heart failure.

Do not misdiagnose my father!

During my argument, which allowed a safe retreat into cardiac-land instead of Daughter-Ville, I threw out a bunch of medical terms and percentages and things beyond their comprehension. It made me feel better for the moment, and I could hear my dad snickering. Mike Dudley was proud of his kids and never failed to let anyone know, in our multiple hospital visits, that I was a nurse. "If you can't get that IV, just let my daughter do it. She's a nurse."

During one VA hospital ICU admission, after Dad's carotid endarterectomy, the nurse popped her head in at the beginning of her shift. She said, "Let me know if you need anything," and never looked in on my dad again. I stayed awake all night watching him, knowing that he was in danger of having a post-surgical stroke if any piece of clot traveled to his brain. Finding safety in the role of a nurse, I paid attention to every detail of his medical progress.

I had arrived at the hospital late for that surgery. Dad was still in pre-op holding, and although he said he did not want anyone to come, I did not listen. He looked at me, and with a tear rolling down his cheek, said, "I knew you'd come. You always do." Dad made me promise to take care of Mama if anything happened to him, and I did. I had never seen my dad cry, and during a moment when he was helpless and full of fear, his only concern was for Mama.

In the morning, when the day shift nurse came into Dad's room, he pointed to my leg and asked me what happened. It was only then that I realized I had removed all of my gel-nails (fake) and had lined them up in order, along the length of my thigh. I do not remember doing it. Maybe the conflict between daughter and nurse created enough anxiety to require an expressive outlet, and my nails gladly sacrificed themselves.

There were so many images, floods of memories, and conflicting feelings. I pushed them down and walked into the house to see my Mama. She told me that she and my dad had sat in the kitchen at about 0100, had coffee, and went to bed in their separate rooms (dad snored). In the morning, Mom made bacon, and when the smell did not wake my dad, Mom went to check on him and found him dead.

She called EMS, who found signs of lividity, indicating he had been dead for several hours. They did not perform CPR. They called their medical authority for permission to declare Dad dead.

Then after calming Mama, they called me.

I do not remember seeing any of them. I do not remember talking to my mom, although I am sure I hugged her and tried not to cry. It upset Mama to see her kids cry, so we tried not to blubber around her. I do remember leaving the house and going to the funeral home because the funeral director said I could come and see my dad and say goodbye if I wanted.

I can still see his face and remember standing over him. I talked to him, I pushed his hair aside, and I told him I loved him. I leaned down and hugged him. When I looked up, I saw the funeral director out of the corner of my eye looking impatient, and then he said something to me that indicated my time was up.

He must have had an appointment, or perhaps having a family say goodbye was so commonplace to him that he did not see the need to give me all the time I needed. My heart broke. This Marine was my Dad, and anyone who has buried a parent understands that it takes more than three minutes to say goodbye.

Mama stayed home from the funeral. She had said her goodbyes, and the memory of finding Dad dead was still too fresh. My brother David stayed with her at the house. Many family members I had not seen in years came. Although they did not know my older siblings well, they knew little Sherry, because I had always been at my dad's side.

When I was involved in a high-speed rollover some years before, I called Dad first, and when the hospital released me, Dad came to take me home. When Dad's best friend died, I showed up at the funeral unannounced, greeted with, "I knew you'd come." On this day, for the last trip Dad and I would take together, I was one of his pallbearers, and stayed with him until the last possible moment.

My dad taught me patriotism, duty, honor, and service; I grew up wanting to be John Wayne. Dad taught me that freedom was anything but free, insisting that I play the Marines Hymn on my clarinet, especially after he had consumed a few beers. Being a Marine was Dad's connection to something bigger than himself, and I took up that baton of servant leadership in any way I could.

We shared pride and appreciation for those who serve in uniform and what the uniform represented. The best I could do was serving in the uniforms of paramilitary and emergency services. As a medic, I cringed when I saw sloppy uniforms of those who failed to realize that they were part of a corps. Their uniforms represent more than the company issuing their paycheck.

Functioning professionally as a medic/RN, and being the family member of someone in need of medical care are opposite sides of the same mirror. As professionals, we can dispassionately see inside to acknowledge the dark places, the little rooms for those in crisis. When we are on the suffering side of the mirror, we can see only our pain reflected in distorted images.

Because we know both sides of the mirror and sometimes step through it, we are aware that in crises, we exist in a world of shadows. We know the sunshine and a different reality exist somewhere, but for those painful moments of loss, we forget how to get there. We need someone to take us by the hand and lead us back into the warmth and cleansing of the sun. We need our support systems to help bring us back from the abyss, because no matter how tough we are, no matter how strong, no matter how smart or talented, and no matter how much we kick and scream that we do not need anyone, we sometimes cannot make it alone.

We all have different reasons for loving or hating what we do, and those reasons may change from day to day. It all comes down to perspective and attitude, and you will find a lot of attitudes in ER, EMS, public safety, and public service personnel. I think the variety of experience, unpredictability of situations, and general fascination with how people think, feel, and act keeps us on our toes. We certainly do not tolerate boredom very well, and if you do not fill our time we will, from both sides of the gurney.

Some of My Favorite Things

I have a theory that a lot of us might be a little ADD (Attention Deficit Disorder). We like challenges, we thrive on variety, and even though we stand strong for our patients as caregivers and advocates, we do not want to see the same people every day. My grandfather said it best about his grandchildren: "Love to see them come, love to see them go." Translation: we like to see something/someone different every couple of hours, or we get bored.

God help any of us behind a desk because we would probably change everyone's font to Wingdings, disable their touchpads, or rearrange files according to the name of the client's pets. You will find me under "Izzy, Honey Dew, or Candy Cane" depending on the day and my mood, and if the filing system is for current or former pet-children.

We have our rituals and superstitions. We do not say the "Q" word (quiet) or the "S" word (slow), because we will cause all "H-E-Double-Hockey-Sticks" to break loose. In EMS, we do not wait if we have to go to the bathroom because waiting will cause a priority-one call (like CPR in progress, major motor vehicle accident, and so on).

We do not take our boots off (yes, you can sleep in them; it takes practice). If we do, the same Gods of EMS will know and tap the dispatcher on the shoulder to send our rig out to BFE (Bum F— Egypt, somewhere very far away). Heaven forbid we order food, because as soon as it arrives, so will a gang shooting with multiple victims, or a house fire, guaranteed.

We prefer not to work on the day of a full moon, or when the brand-spanking-new residents go from short coat to long coat as they transition from medical student to doctor. Both situations are bad, and there are no incantations, scented candles, or massage oils that will alter one's fate under those circumstances. Getting back to the original statement about ADD and challenges and the oddities of folks who do what we do, I must admit that I love all of those things.

I suppose you could say that I am a neo-Freudian cognitive behaviorist who peeks into Plato's Cave, buys chew toys for Pavlov's dog, and may occasionally toss Ayurvedistic smoke bombs toward staunch practitioners of the oh-so-sacred scientific method while skipping down Pollyanna Lane toward the Mecca of postmodern psychology and positivism.

Perhaps we are a group that demonstrates a portion of the Peter Pan Principle. We do not want to grow up. Dealing with life and death encourages our wanting to play a little harder than the average bear. My son-in-law Scott is a firefighter medic, as are many friends and family, and they are a unique breed. Have you ever heard of grown men having Nerf Wars indoors? I have pictures.

Entire rooms in our homes are dedicated to artists' images and souvenirs of what we do because we are proud. Tasteful shrines to our professions are acceptable. Becoming Joe Medic or Joe Firefighter with stickers and portable light bars, and walking around town in scrubs "because they are comfortable" is not. Nor is it desirable to become a walking caricature of Nancy Nurse with little embroidered hearts sewn on your non-work socks and shoes.

Some things are just downright embarrassing.

~ ~ ~

Random thoughts: I wonder what was going through the mind of the person who once called our ambulance service and asked a favor. It seems that the sirens of passing ambulances disturbed parishioners during church services. The caller wanted to know if we could please turn the sirens off when in the vicinity of the church, although lights were ok because they did not bother anyone inside the building.

My answer had something to do with legal and safety concerns. I was polite, but I wanted to ask if she was freaking kidding me. It did not seem an appropriate Christian response.

I wonder if the well-dressed good-looking man whose car was assaulted by a deer (yes, the deer ran into him) was as embarrassed by my performing a physical head to toe assessment on him as I was while doing it. I was a newbie, and there was nothing wrong with the fellow. My partner Nelda, an experienced medic, insisted on the transport. Nelda giggled on the drive to the hospital. I think it was a newbie-initiation setup.

As I advanced from EMT to EMTS, and finally to EMTP (paramedic) in charge, I wondered if I would know what calls I could handle. When should I call for help? When my partner and I responded to a car that hit a large dirt pile at a high rate of speed, leaped 20 feet in the air taking out tree branches, and then ejected both the driver and passenger, I had my answer. As I walked toward the patient impaled by a tree branch I realized that yep, it was pretty much a no-brainer. We called for backup.

I wonder how much of this gallows humor folks who read this book will understand, appreciate, and accept as part of our coping mechanisms without taking offense. For example, former ER Resident Pete quotes our beloved ER doc DB, who remarked, immediately after smoothly intubating a drug overdose patient, "I've never lost a chemical war yet." The ES folks understand, and if you are a Trauma Junkie, that is pretty funny.

~ ~ ~

The first time I had a woman in my trauma center acute care module presenting with recent symptoms of a stroke, I did not jump up and down declaring I knew what to do and would perform a miracle. Truthfully, I switched into autopilot and busied myself performing standard patient care protocol steps. It gave my brain a few minutes to catch up to the situation. The scenario plays itself out with different patients on different days, but the goal of good care is the same regardless of the patient or medical complaint.

I hook the patient to the monitor and oxygen while telling the secretary I need a doctor *now* (we rarely use *stat*). I ask the tech to get an EKG and start two IVs while simultaneously drawing blood for the gazillion tests in the algorithm. Of course, the crackerjack secretary, who is also familiar with the protocols, is entering orders into the computer for a head CT and lab work simultaneously as she phones the doctor.

On this day, I ask all of the pertinent questions of the patient while trying to calm her and her family members. I bond with her in a way that reassures her that we work calmly but fast. I tell her that many things will happen to her very quickly.

One side of her face is drooping, and one side of her body is flaccid. The symptoms started shortly before the patient arrived, so I know there is hope if we enter into warp drive and get everything done. I begin filling out the consent forms in preparation for special procedures and medications.

It all happens in a flash. The sickening recognition that things could go blissfully right or terribly wrong hang over my head like a dark cloud. The medication used to treat an acute CVA (Cerebrovascular Accident, or stroke) can improve or almost completely resolve symptoms. Or it can cause further damage.

We consult a list of inclusion and exclusion criteria before using the medication. It is called tPA (tissue plasminogen activator, or clot buster). Located in the magic tPA box, which is just a small, plastic, brightly colored toolbox from a discount hardware store, is everything one needs to perform this particular miracle.

The doctor evaluates, the appropriate sister departments run and result their tests, and the nurse using protocol-based criterion administers the medication. Then we wait. The first time I used this drug, back before stroke teams responded to an acute CVA, was one of the greatest ER moments I can remember.

The patient could not talk. One side of her body was completely limp. While looking into my eyes, she shed a tear that broke my heart. Fear, trust, and hope lived behind that single tear. Amid all the fuss and bother, I gently squeezed the hand on my side of the bed (the arm with the IVs through which I was carefully administering her medications) and tried to deliver words of encouragement.

The tPA protocol involves making regular re-assessments of the patient's function. It was not long before this patient could not only move her affected arm and leg but also lift the formerly flaccid arm high enough to reach and tenderly touch, with the lightest grace of her fingertips, the face of her husband, who stood supportively at her side. She looked at me and spoke her first words, almost surprised that they came out so clearly. She whispered a "thank you" that I can still hear. It probably did not help matters that she reminded me of my Mama, or maybe that is why I fought a little harder, prayed a little more, and remember her still.

This sweet little person in a bathrobe with snow-white hair and soulful eyes was a beautiful picture of overcoming obstacles and beating enormously unfavorable odds. We have more sorrows than joys in ER and EMS. Saves and successes are not as plentiful as we would like. This particular victory will live in my heart long after I put down my stethoscope for the last time.

~ ~ ~

Earlier, I introduced you to Uncle Randy, one of the youngsters I worked with early in my paramedic career. I adore the young fellow. He is not much older than my son Christopher and is one of those clean-cut respectful kids you want to bring home to meet your family, trust with the key to your house, and offer the combination to your safe. These reasons and more are why I love to give Uncle Randy (as my daughter Missy calls him) a hard time. Only family can pick on family.

When Randy and I worked at the same volunteer EMS service, we did not have the opportunity to work together very often. On one particular call, when Randy and I were in separate ambulances, he called for backup, and I responded. Randy had a seizing patient in an old farmhouse. The place was dark, and Randy was trying to stabilize the patient to get an IV so he could administer the appropriate medications. I told Randy to radio the hospital for the med orders, and I would get the IV.

The older man was lying on his back in the middle of the living room with his daughter sitting on the floor next to him. I got my equipment ready, and then directed the daughter to hold her father's legs down as best she could while I worked on the IV. I sat on the floor with my feet facing the man's head, wrapped my legs around his convulsing arm to hold it still, and secured an IV in his forearm.

It was not the most graceful IV start I have ever done, but in retrospect, it was one of the most challenging, and therefore, the most fun. Randy never questioned my tennis shoe prints on the man's shoulder. He simply administered the medication, stabilized his patient, and delivered him safely to the hospital. It is no wonder that medics sometimes laugh at folks who cannot find a vein to draw blood or start an IV in clean, well-lit, controlled environments.

Can I get a Hoo-Ah, Fist Pump, or High Five?

~ ~ ~

Life is not all glitz and glamour in emergency services. We run into folks who want, without benefit of formal training, to be the next John Gage or Roy Desoto (*Emergency*, 1970s). Some unlicensed folks buy gear bags and keep them in their trunks without the first clue of what to do with their equipment. They think because they have watched television showing dramatic reenactments of emergencies that they are qualified to administer emergency care, itching to be first on scene at an accident so they can be the Good Samaritan who saves a life.

I was in a long line of cars on the Arizona side of the Hoover Dam once when a fellow got out of his car and started walking the mile to an accident scene. The dude was newly into an EMT class, so fancied that he was obligated to respond. As he passed by my convertible, I asked a few questions and discovered he did not have so much as a pair of gloves. This man wearing open sandals and shorts had not yet heard about universal precautions, scene safety, and not getting in over your head. He turned around and walked back to his car. The imagined vision of heroic deeds and thankful citizens is often just so much Hollywood scripting.

When you wear the uniform and take home the whopping paycheck of a professional emergency services worker, or even if you volunteer and get only a stipend, the game changes. Those who do this work sometimes have moments when we *do* feel like a hero, times when we know that we have made a difference. There are dues we pay for those moments. Sometimes we pay emotionally with large denomination bills, and other times we toss nickels at minor annoyances that come with the territory.

When I was a medic du jour down in the city during nursing school, I might have a different partner/city/ambulance every weekend. One station was next to a hospital: a one-bedroom apartment with a bunkroom, living room, two large couches, TV, full kitchen, and access to a washer and dryer. Folks dreamed about such luxury, and even though we rarely slept in those quarters (24-hour shifts did not guarantee any time for sleep), we sometimes knew the joys of a home-cooked microwave dinner.

One of our stations was a little less comfortable. The main living area was a single room without air-conditioning (blistering summers), with two twin beds and a single bathroom. If you wanted to shower, you had to walk outside and enter (at your own risk) into a single stall that one dare not use with bare feet. The attached ambulance bay was much nicer, with room for two rigs, a supply area, and equipment to wash the ambulances.

During summer shifts, one lost all inhibitions. When returning to quarters, even if the crew was male/female, exhausted and overheated medics might strip down to their t-shirts and shorts and lie on top of their bedrolls. We usually enjoyed only a few minutes of fitful sleep before the next call came from dispatch.

They called me "Bagel B—ch." We never knew if or when we might drive through a fast-food restaurant, so I often carried bagels in my backpack, with a frozen two-liter bottle of flavored water so I would have something cold to drink (it slowly melted). Through nursing school, I lived on "B" foods: Bean Burritos, Bananas, and Blueberry Bagels. EMS and ER folks carry extra provisions in their backpacks because you may work more than a single 24-hour shift, so having extra food, clothing, and hygiene supplies on hand is smart.

One of my three jobs was at a volunteer station in a small town in the thumb area of Michigan. The EMS quarters and ambulance bay were part of the police station, and there were two possible places to sleep. The first was the nice bunkroom that had a fridge, microwave, coffee pot, and bunk beds. The other housed an old, filthy carpet, and unwelcome roommates (mice) in the couch placed across from the television.

Whenever I worked with "Uncle Randy," he would invariably arrive first and grab the bunks leaving me with the dirty TV room. EMS is without chivalry. We volunteers received a stipend for on-call shifts, and I sometimes worked more than 30 12-hour shifts in a month. There was a shower in the fire station next door, but the fire chief would not allow me, a female, to use *his* facility, even if no one was in the building. EMS is so glamorous!

A joyful highlight of working City EMS is something called "sitting cover." When the ambulances take calls and move out of their assigned areas, the dispatchers will move other ambulances around to cover their territory. Unfortunately, that means that if you got to sleep at 0300 and you are the "last car" available, you might have to get out of bed and drive the ambulance to a point a few miles away. When the other ambulance comes back in service, if you have not gotten a call, you may get to return to bed.

Honestly, this is how many folks learn to sleep sitting up, even with lights flashing and sirens blaring. It may also explain why being called to a party store at 0400 for someone who has a headache from drinking all night and wants a ride home may be a little off-putting. Your medic may not be as pleasant or sympathetic as you feel they should be under the circumstances.

A firefighter-medic told me recently that taking 13 to 17 calls in a 24-hour shift keeps him busy, but as long as they are true medical emergencies, he does not mind. However, there are too many nonsense calls that take ambulances out of service and unavailable for real emergencies. The party store woman with a hangover headache, who wanted the ambulance to take her across town to the hospital near her house, was also expecting a stretcher ride. Sadly, she was quite disappointed with her medics when they walked her into the back of the ambulance and belted her onto the bench seat. I am sure you are not surprised to discover that same patient wanted a cab voucher home from the ER after getting a warm blanket, ice water, medications, prescription for pain pills, and a meal-in-a-box to go.

~ ~ ~

Attitude is everything. Beyond Descartes' "I think, therefore I am," a lot of critical thinking attached to education, skill, and experience precedes the happening of events. For example, starting IVs requires more than knowing procedures; it requires a deft hand and fine understanding of human anatomy. Venipuncture (starting IVs) is an artform. Ask anyone with "rolling veins" or claims that "nobody can ever get an IV on me" the importance of a good poker.

Veins roll more on some people than others partly because folks lose fat and connective tissue that anchors veins in place. Those medical folks who label you at fault because of your rolling veins are probably just not that good. Ask Mindy D.[*] or Kathy B., two of the best nurses and pokers I know, and the only two I would welcome atop this particular soapbox.

We who are good at poking love doing it, and if you say, "Good luck," please do not be surprised to hear us say, "Luck has nothing to do with it. I am very good at what I do. If you do your part, I'll do mine, and together we will get this done as quickly and painlessly as possible."

Patients who are bleeding profusely either internally or externally need two large-bore IVs (great big needles) and fluid replacement, or the empty tank (circulating blood) will cause the pump (heart) to fail. That situation translates to cardiac arrest and a lousy day for the patient and staff. Mindy and I once had a patient who was bleeding internally, so we approached the fellow, one of us on each arm, and in a contest about which the poor fellow was unaware, slid IVs in at the same time. Mission accomplished, patient stabilized, fluid resuscitation initiated, and two nurses with attitude and aptitude mentally high-fiving at the bedside.

~ ~ ~

When a caregiver goes the extra mile to do things beyond his or her job, some patients feel the need to acknowledge that attention. Nurses may stay past the end of shift to deliver a dose of pain medications, so the patient does not have to wait for the oncoming shift to get through report. Nurses may do battle with a newbie resident to get the appropriate medication to relieve a cancer patient's nausea, especially when that patient knows from experience what works and how much it takes.

Sometimes nurses will plead with the doctor in charge to admit patients who cannot take care of themselves but are too proud to ask, as an advocate for patients who need someone to act on their behalf. As a nurse, I have done all of these things as a matter of course. They are small moments but often make a bigger difference to our patients than we realize until we become patients ourselves.

I have had more surgeries than Carter has little pills, so my experience on the other side of the gurney is quite lengthy. I was in a high-speed rollover resulting in hairline fractures of my neck. I doubled over in the middle of my workplace after fighting tummy pain for months (nurses tough it out), winning five itty-bitty scars from a cholecystectomy (gallbladder removal).

During another shift, the docs admitted me for a debilitating heart irregularity that caused shortness of breath, dizziness, diaphoresis (sweating), and weakness. Of course, I had to wait for the charge nurse to find someone to take over for me before I hit the gurney and collapsed (close but no cigar), but that is what nurses and medics do. We push beyond our limits because we place our patients first, even if it means working until we drop.

I have shattered my left ankle (level ground; must have been an earth tremor), broken my left foot, left baby toe, left wrist, left ribs, and dislocated my left elbow (not sure what the left side pattern indicates). Surgeries included all of the female parts, appendix, both feet (plates and screws), both eyes (several times), a new neck (more plates, screws, and donor bone), and some elective stuff.

I am becoming bionic. Medicine has the technology, and none of my plates or screws set off airport metal detectors, so let's go for it. I am quite sure there is more to come, as my lower back, from decades of EMS and ER, requires yet another intervention that I will defer as long as possible. Lumbar discs: gone.

Is there a positive aspect to all of these experiences? Yes. I know what the little things mean when you are hurting, alone, and have no control over your situation. This awareness means that I am not as likely to forget the little things when I take care of you.

I remember the OR tech whose smile I could hear long before I was able to open my eyes. She gave me a most-appreciated bedpan and made no objection when I missed—a little. I remember a tech who gave me a wet washcloth to moisten my lips as I tried (for 24 hours) to push out my preemie firstborn.

I also remember the private duty nurse who forgot to wrap my post-operative areas to reduce swelling and bruising, and the noise she made with her medic assistant at the desk outside my room all night. I was their only patient and paid out of pocket for them to take care of me. I saw them only once during the long night, and they continued to chatter loudly about personal things while in the room with me. I learned what not to do.

Because of bad experiences as a patient, I understand gratitude after good care. Patients may want to return the kindness, but good care should be the rule rather than the exception. One former patient owned a seasonal ice cream parlor and wanted me to stop by for a free container when they opened in the spring. The genuine appreciation and kind words were enough, and I remember them because they welcomed me into their lives and allowed me to share in a positive outcome. Genuine appreciation is much better than ice cream.

~ ~ ~

There are various levels of competency in all segments of medicine, and those of us who have a minimal level of training and functional capability have expectations. We hope for the best and prepare for the worst, but when care of our loved ones is involved, we will not tolerate ignorance. We can all appreciate that folks who successfully obtain medical licensure are not idiots. One must be relatively intelligent to pass required licensing boards.

Nevertheless, passing tests does not immediately confer wisdom. Nor does it confirm an ability to think critically, and it certainly does not portend any level of common sense. Common sense and competency are on my list of favorite things, but sometimes they are hard to find in certain segments of the medical community.

My ex-husband and I discovered the nadir of the rectum of medicine ("Rectum: Wrecked him? Darn near killed him!"). That playful twisting of words had become my nightmare sitting on both the patient and the family member's side of the treatment bed. I prefer the other side of the needle, thank you, where I have some level of informed participation, and of course, control.

We spent a few years as nomads, thinking it was time to slow down and settle into a place of beautiful scenery and a slower pace. We heard it said that walking is what people do between retirement and death. I did a lot of walking until something went bump in the night. We sought medical attention in that nameless area and learned that when their medical folks are good, they are very, very good, but when they are bad, they are horrid.

In the case of the ex, a shoulder problem required, in my opinion, minimal testing and a referral to an orthopedic specialist. Instead, the small-town doc decided that physical therapy and magic potions, lotions, and massages were a better idea. I silently fumed, knowing the protocols for his complaint. He who knew nothing medical (ex) decided to give the doctor and physical therapist a chance, and I nearly bit through my lip. I can still feel the scar tissue.

Eight weeks after starting the wand-waving, without improving, my ex received his long-requested referral to an orthopod (orthopedic doctor). The orthopod was intelligent and current with professional literature, a shining gem displaying the humility of a man who does not need to stomp his feet in authority. Ex got two shots of steroids and canceled further unnecessary physical therapy.

My experience in BFE involved a long runaround with that same primary doc who unnecessarily changed my medications (I gained 20 pounds), giving me stuff I knew from the literature did not work. He denied the need for additional tests after films showed irregularities but stopped my hormone replacement therapy, and recommended vitamin D.

I shared my concerns with a small group of close friends (support systems!). The lack of hormones, hot flashes, sleeplessness, and all the other fun stuff, including unspoken fears, continued for several months until we moved back to the land of good medicine. The beautiful word "benign" (thank you Dr. Cheryl W.) set my mind at ease, and I am on an appropriate schedule for follow-up testing.

And now we return to the other side of the gurney.

We ES folks are patient advocates. We have a general idea of what needs to happen, and we respectfully pursue those avenues. Sometimes we are not so delicate about it (my son-in-law Scott has been asked to leave certain medical facilities after fighting for appropriate care for his wife, Michele, and dog, Gracie). We cannot tolerate ignorance. If you see steam rising from our ears, it is because someone has just said or done something so incredibly inappropriate or inconceivably ignorant that a rubber band snaps in our brains. It hurts.

The advice is this: educate yourselves. Do not accept every word from every medical professional as gospel. Sometimes overzealous patients and family members drive medical folk nuts with their internet searches and suggested medical myths and potions, but ask for information. You have a right to have things explained to you in a way you understand.

Ask medical professionals for their rationale ("why"), ask about current research, and ask about their plan of action. If anyone pats you on the hand and answers with, "because *I* am the doctor, *I* went to medical school, you did not, and you have to trust me," then *run*. Sometimes you are the only advocate for yourself, friends, or family. Research, talk to trusted and appropriate professionals who are familiar with your type of situation, present your information and questions respectfully but do not permit intimidation.

The awesome orthopod in BFE talked about his efforts to educate local doctors. He also mentioned that some of his biggest obstacles and objections involve doctors who do not listen to their patients. Amen brother, good medical folks are some of my favorite things in life, from both sides of the gurney. Thank you for educating us, for explaining options, for providing information about current practices, and especially for actively caring.

~ ~ ~

We who dance around the ER at the speed of light, often in dizzying circles, have jacket pockets stuffed full of things. We carry hemoccult developer, non-latex gloves, tourniquets, hemostats (several sizes), and extra pens (the communicable diseases patients keep pens used to sign discharge papers and consent forms). We stuff slips of paper marked with patients' names, room numbers, reports, and pertinent notes. There are extra paper clips (to hang IV bags from odd places), and at least four sizes of angiocaths (IV needles).

In our clean pocket, we store an emergency bag of peanut M&Ms (who eats?), a sterile urine cup (never one handy when you need it), and post-it notes (to give patients their latest vital signs). I long ago abandoned trying to keep things organized, and settled for a "dirty pocket, clean pocket" system in the jacket tied to my waist. The filled pockets knocked into things as I ran through the ER, sometimes hooking on errant hall stretchers. The back pocket of my scrubs was for cash, though we rarely carried more than we needed to buy lunch or specialty coffee from the vendor just outside the ER doors.

What doesn't fit in our pockets but seems to find a permanent place in our hearts are the folks who make us realize that we are human. We are fallible, and we cannot keep everyone at a professional distance. We never know when someone will enter our hearts, or in what way, and what we will do with those feelings when the shift is over, and we go home to a silence that allows thoughts to enter our awareness.

Today I thought about a patient I had years ago, a woman who was dying, who should have died hours before. I had no idea what to do about her, as I had spent hours on the phone trying to get some family members to come in and say goodbye. The charge nurse came into the patient's cubicle, leaned down, and brushing fine wisps of hair from the elderly woman's forehead said, "You don't have to fight anymore, Grandma. It's OK to go. It is time to go." It was not long until the woman took her last breath.

We are Trauma Junkies with incredibly well-developed trauma armor. Sometimes that armor cracks, and there is only so much duct tape. That experienced nurse reminded me that sometimes the kindest thing is to help folks let go.

~ ~ ~

Jumping back and forth across both sides of the gurney can be confusing. Sometimes we ES folks are so geeked by the unusual that we hardly mind, or notice for that matter, that we continually flop around between family, caregiver, rescuer and patient roles. The most recent example of such confusion happened not long ago as I prepared for bed. It was 2100 (9 p.m.), and I had just taken a bedtime dose of Benadryl seconds before the phone rang.

Missy: "Mom, my water broke."

Me: "Fix it. Put it back. I just took Benadryl. You cannot go into labor right now."

Missy showered, and I threw some street clothes on while a super-strong mega-caffeine brain-jolting K-cup brewed from the Keurig. Coffee in hand, I headed out the door driving the 0.38 miles to Missy's house. Missy's husband Scott was on duty, as Missy was not due to for inducement until Tuesday. This was Friday night. Missy called the station, found out that Scott was on a rescue call working a cardiac arrest (of course!). The Battalion Chief radioed Scott and immediately sent another medic to relieve him.

Our ride progressed until we saw the sky light up with flashing lights. Sirens whined, and expressway traffic hastily slowed to a crawl. We would not escape a bit of drama; a car on the side of the road was fully engulfed in flames. Missy grabbed her cell phone and snapped a picture of the inferno that had no regard for a woman in labor (we needed proof: who would believe us?). Escaping a road soon blocked by emergency vehicles and rubbernecking gawkers who crashed into one another behind us, we drove on.

As I started to turn into the hospital, I saw a car in my rearview mirror traveling at a high rate of speed, so I waited to see if the driver might like to get past us. He did. The car swerved wildly, cut me off, and screeched to a halt in front of us at the ER entrance. Passengers jumped out of all four doors screaming, and ER staff ran toward the car with a stretcher. Scott was waiting at the ER door, and we saw him heading to assist with removing a stabbing victim from the car.

Scott provided a textbook example of how we keep jumping across that proverbial gurney.

I hollered, Scott saw us, switched from paramedic mode to husband/father mode, and headed back for a wheelchair. I parked the car and prepared for a very long night waiting for the birth, reminding myself that I was not a Paramedic RN that night. I was Missy's Mumma. Andrew Rhys made his grand entrance the next morning, and he could not be more perfect. He has his mother's eyes.

~ ~ ~

Sometimes our professional and personal worlds collide. It has taken many years to discuss the following experience; it ripped my heart out then and still hurts now. Honey was a Cocker Spaniel who walked into my life, and my car, after her previous family unceremoniously dumped her at the side of the road. When my ex-husband bounced me down the stairs and out of my house, I had nowhere to put Honey. Eventually my son Christopher, who also had a blonde Cocker named TJ, welcomed her. Honey and TJ lived with 'Topher while I finished nursing school and looked for my own home.

Honey, TJ, and Caesar

The day Honey came into our lives, I determined not to let her own me. I called her "Honey" as you might refer to someone generically as "Dear" or "Sweetie." Her thick blonde hair, covered in burrs from being out in the fields, did little to hide her scrawny frame. I was not going to bring that mess into my home, so I spent the afternoon cutting away those probably painful attachments. Honey looked up at me as if to say, "I trust you with my life," and never flinched.

We asked around town, made the appropriate calls, but could not find her owner. Folks laughed at me for even trying, saying she was dumped on Monday, the day the stockyards opened for bringing in livestock and visiting the large open-air market. Many pets found themselves homeless and alone on Mondays because those who did the dropping assumed someone, possibly local farmers who had plenty of room, would adopt them.

Honey was about two years old and soon took over my heart. She had the healing qualities of most animals, serving up generous portions of unconditional love, and becoming my closest friend and confidante. While we lived in that small town, I had acquaintances but few friends until I joined the local volunteer EMS. Even then, there were things you did not tell your fellow workers, but you could confide in your dog. Maybe Honey is the reason having a pet as a support system post-crisis made so much sense to me when I read studies about pet therapy.

The kids, Topher and Missy, both loved Honey, and she thrived in their presence. Our home life was not without challenges as the marriage slowly worked toward a terminal end, but Honey was a comfort and joy for the three of us. She considered herself so much an equal part of our family that when we went away for a weekend, the folks who came in to feed her noticed she would not eat unless one of them ate something. She was socialized and part human.

Honey did not take too kindly to monthly abandonment at the groomer, defiantly peeing on the hardwood floors after returning home from her haircuts. I learned to hold her reassuringly in my arms for half an hour after each grooming, telling her how beautiful she was, and that we loved her. We adapted with "summer cuts," reducing groomer visits, leaving only those beautiful floppy ears as identifying the shorn blonde a Cocker Spaniel.

Several years later, divorced, with nursing school completed, and looking for a full-time hospital job, I continued to work EMS. Topher had his own home in the city, and his Cocker Spaniel, TJ (Topher Junior). Honey came to live with TJ and Topher because she was too rambunctious to stay with Missy and me at my parents' house. We saw it as a temporary arrangement while I continued to look for a new job and home.

I visited TJ and Honey when I worked the city EMS job, still living up in the boonies with my parents. Missy and I shared a sparse room in my parents' home. While not ideal, it gave Missy extra time with Grandpa, who died 3 ½ years after we moved out. I remember riding in the ambulance and looking at the smallest gatehouses thinking, "We could live there. We could make that work." My paramedic salary was not enough to support even a small apartment, and my heart longed for the three of us, me, Missy, and Honey, to be together.

One weekend while working the city ambulance job, I received a frantic call from my son. He was trying to tell me that Honey was sick. She was seizing, and he was driving her to an animal hospital only a few minutes from my assigned station. We had just delivered a patient to the ER, and I was waiting for my partner to finish writing her report. I called the supervisor, telling him I needed to go to the vet's office, and he said he would get back with me.

I waited for what seemed like an eternity. Precious time passed while Honey waited for her Mumma to come.

Several calls later, from son Topher, and from me to the EMS supervisor, I received permission to drive the short distance to the vet's office, which was in our coverage area. When I walked in, the female vet ushered Topher and me into a private room. I rejected her words as my knees buckled, and I dropped onto the seat behind me. I heard that horrible sound, the stifled scream of loss that I had heard so many times on the road and in the hospital when someone died. It took a moment to realize it was not the animals around me making that noise.

It was coming from me.

I held Honey in my arms while she seized and told the vet to make it stop. Stop her suffering, as I could not bear to see her hurting. Normally, the vet told me, there is paperwork required before administering a lethal injection. The vet, crying along with Topher and me, decided to set formality aside and hurriedly prepared the injection. I held Honey closely, patted her short, fresh, summer haircut, and told her how beautiful she was. Telling her I loved her, and how sorry I was, I felt her seizing stop and her body become limp in my arms. I kissed her little face for the last time.

Honey had found loose coins on the floor in Topher's home and ingested them. The metal in the coins is toxic, especially to small dogs, and the heavy metal toxicity (Richardson, Gwatlney-Brant, & Villar, 2002) caused Honey's irreversible seizures and led to her death. After signing all of the papers, I put Honey's body, lying in a cardboard coffin-shaped white box, in the back of the ambulance and called our rig out of service. I needed to take Honey home.

My partner said little to me on the ride back to our station. She knew there were no words, and even though she and I had dealt with death more times than we could remember, this was different. As medics, we stood challenging death daily, and when we lost the battle, we went on to fight again. There was no fight left in me that day. I put Honey in the back of my car and drove the 130 miles, sobbing all the way home with a broken heart that still defies mending.

The next day I put Honey somewhere I thought she would be happy, a place she might have chosen herself. Honey loved to sleep with her bum (Canadian for buttocks) up against things (me especially). Once, after a visit to the home of my dear friend Deb (a fellow ER nurse) and her black Cocker Spaniel, Caesar, Deb told me Caesar had started sleeping with his bum up against her face. She asked me to tell Honey to stop channeling through Caesar!

Honey's coffin sat with her back comfortably against a fallen log in a large wooded area of my sister's yard. I have never been back there. I can no more visit Honey's grave than I can the cemetery housing my Dad's coffin. I do not want to remember that part of our lives.

I think those of us who face the types of things that people should never see, much less bear responsibility for, sometimes know our limitations. We cannot change the bad things that happen. We cannot stop things from going bump in the night. We have little control beyond our professional toys with their bright colors, lights, bells, and whistles.

In our personal lives, I think sometimes we are so full of "crazy" that there is no more room. There is no diversionary, protocol-following place to escape to when we are not in uniform. We cannot emotionally remove ourselves, or over-intellectualize, or employ common professional-duty coping mechanisms. We have nowhere to run, and we cannot get away from ourselves.

When bad things happen to those we love, we hurt. If we cannot change the cause of the hurt, if we have no solid way to make it better, then we stuff it. We bury it. We refuse to look at it, and if it threatens to resurface, we expend all of our time and energy pushing it down again. It takes enormous energy to present images of normalcy, keeping others from seeing our pain or weakness, and by golly, we pull and play those cards far too often. We need a new deck.

Put me in the middle of a crisis, and I busy myself following algorithms and watching measurable changes take place. Give me an impossible situation, and I will delight in finding a way to solve it, to find or create answers where none existed before. Give me someone dying, and I am your medical and emotional rock. Let something happen to those I love, take away hope, and I am lost. Sometimes when every breath hurts, even though your support systems are near, nothing helps more than time.

Please understand that I am not comparing animals to humans. For many of us, the animals *are* our family, and we love them dearly. They help us cope, they entertain us, they give us peace, and in my case especially, they help us heal. During a CISM (Critical Incident Stress Management) post-incident group intervention, we always ask about support systems, which include our four-footed family members.

I remember the examples demonstrated by Dr. Joan Coughlin, PsyD, a certified thanatologist (grief and loss specialist dealing with death-related issues), who led our crisis response out-briefings after Katrina. She did not ask "if" folks had anyone at home to talk to, she asked "who" folks had to talk to when they got home from their disaster service. She made a point to include pets as support systems, and the light bulbs going off above heads in the room nearly blinded us. Folks will confide in their pets and take comfort from them. Sometimes there are no words, or the words are those you might not trust to just anyone. Talk to your pets.

I have learned a lot, including how a ministry of presence, in silence, can comfort the wounded. I have felt the unconditional love from my four-footed children and grandchildren, and have become a staunch defender of those who understand their value. They are our family, so if someone loses a beloved pet, please do not dismiss his or her grief with "it was only an animal."

Honey, TJ, and Caesar thank you.

POSTMORTEM

If anything in this section touched your heart, thank you for sitting with me through recounting some very personal moments. The hurt never goes away. It changes, and grief evolves, when we process it, to a way of remembering without falling apart. We never get over it, we get through it.

Rereading means reliving, which can be quite painful, especially for Empaths and Highly Sensitive People (HSP). Often people like me are criticized for being "too sensitive," usually by those who are flinging emotional poo and do not want to face responsibility. Sensitivity becomes an insult, wounding words to point out perceived imperfections. Being empathetic is not a fault, but Empaths do need to take precautions to remain internally safe.

HSPs sometimes intentionally avoid violent movies, TV shows, and the news. They can be overwhelmed by bright lights, coarse fabrics, strong smells, and piercing noises like sirens. Sometimes they need to walk away from overwhelming situations and chaos into darkened or private places to reduce the stimuli. They may prioritize activities to avoid drama and can be rattled or overwhelmed by too many tasks. Teachers may have commented that they were shy children with internal complexities.

How many nurses do you know who refuse to watch the news (for various expressed reasons), perhaps saying, "I get enough of that at work?" How many are deemed distant or antisocial for not participating in loud parties and get-togethers? How many are great at work until they get to a certain point and then either lose it or say, "I have to walk away for a minute?" Not all of us are HSP; if you are, give yourself a break (and read about HSPs), if you know someone who may be, don't judge (and read about HSPs).

So why do sensitive people get into public service or emergency response? They care, sometimes too much, and sometimes do not see the edge of the cliff until they topple over. In caring for others, boundaries are necessary to keep us emotionally safe, yet not always possible to maintain. If something hits too close to home (a familiar face, circumstance, perfume, piece of clothing), we can lose our distance as our boundaries falter. We bleed emotionally with a smile on our faces because people expect us to be strong, and we do not want to disappoint.

I miss my Dad (and now Mama) every day. If someone reminds me of them, I may completely lose it once alone. If you ask me to talk about Honey, TJ, and Caesar, I can for about 30 seconds of fact revelation, and then the pain hits. My throat tightens, my eyes threaten to tear, and I have to change the subject, take a deep breath, and silence the inner screams.

And that's the problem many of us face; we still try to maintain a "tough enough" exterior. I was not that tough when I met the state troopers and coroner in my Dad's driveway, when I cared for that sweet woman who had a stroke (I can still hear that "Thank you" and see her face), or when we lost our puppies.

Over the past few decades, I have taught many Critical Incident Stress Management courses all around the continental US and Alaska. I believe that people who put their lives and emotional wellbeing on the line deserve to know how to deal with the emotional aftermath of trauma, to deal with the known and often experienced emotional reactions to seeing, smelling, doing what people should not see, smell, do. Police, fire, EMS, ER -- some need a minor boost in their coping and resilience skill toolsets. Some are close to the edge.

"Please take care of each other and yourselves" is the same song I've been singing since 1989, the one thing that, in retrospect, has not changed.

Part IV

Ah... Memories

EMS calls and ER situations are not always drama and tragedy. Under the right circumstances, we have an absolute blast, usually because we are somewhat in control of often-uncontrollable situations. When those moments happen, when we get to do our jobs well without incident and have positive outcomes, we are geeked. Other memorable calls are not always medically successful but remain with us because we are welcomed into the most private and personal inner circles of family.

This next section blends EMS and ER because even though we wear different uniforms, we are essentially different arms of the same body. Working for multiple agencies, sometimes we have to look down at our uniforms to see who or what we are that day. When I was in nursing school, I worked in a hospital ER and with two EMS agencies. If I woke up suddenly I grabbed my covers: if I was in a sleeping bag, it was EMS. If I had a regular blanket, I was at home. Either way, waking from deep sleep to some obnoxious noise meant addressing something emergent that could involve life or death. No wonder many of us are hypervigilant and addicted to caffeine.

~ ~ ~

Having a calm, confident EMS partner who knows the rules and protocols, is especially competent with his skills, loves to teach, and treats you with the respect of a big brother makes a 24-hour shift fly by. Bob T. was one of those big brothers and still buoys me with positive words that mean more than I can express. I asked Bob if he remembered a call we'd responded to over 15 years ago, and surprisingly, he did. Bob writes, "I bragged to everyone who would listen how wonderful my partner Sherry was because she knew sign language, and saved the day. You rocked in EMS." My heart is still swelling, and being able to step out from the shadows to "rock" and "save the day" reflect childhood dreams of growing up and being a hero, even if only for a moment.

Bowling, Anyone?

Working the city of Joseph Park* was fun, mostly because we had a good relationship with the firefighters, and it did not hurt that there were several places to eat nearby if you had the time for a meal. In that area, if we had a firefighter third rider, certain departments budgeted to pay for the crew's meal, a definite benefit when your salary tops out at $9.53/hr. Our 24-hour shifts were feast or famine, but because I was somewhat familiar with the area and usually had a good partner, I loved that station, especially when they were medic-medic. Putting two equally licensed partners together was a luxury in Warwick County* because the legal requirement called for medic-specialist (EMTP and EMTS), which meant that after stabilizing the patient, the paramedic attended every call and the specialist drove the rig.

Another particularly pleasant prerequisite was that sometimes I got to work with Bob T. Bob eventually joined the enemy (administration), but when I partnered with him, Bob was a working medic with the additional duty assignment of white-shirted Field Training Officer (FTO). FTOs and administration are color-coded (white shirts) to separate them from the working-class stiffs. We knew that white shirts represented white flags: surrender your nonsensical ways when they appear, follow the rules, do not mess around.

I internalized a healthy fear of making a mistake in front of supervisors and authority figures. I also bore an incredible sense of urgency that produced such a high level of stress. I fried out a few otherwise healthy organs. Working with Bob T. brought a sense of calm.

My heart still raced at the sound of the tones dispatching us to something-somewhere-out-there, and I hungered to know more about what I was doing. Some medics traveled with color-coded cards outlining pre and post radio contact algorithms and treatment protocols. I barely had time to skim over my nursing school reading, so always appreciated experienced partners.

As I recall, when Bob and I received the dispatch to the LightningBowl* bowling alley, it was a deceptively warm and carefree day. With mid-day calls, there is no anticipation of tragedy, and that is when things may catch you off guard. If the moon is full, or you are mid-snowstorm, you expect and prepare for the worst, appreciating anything less. We were going to a bowling alley, anticipated a twisted ankle, thumb stuck in a bowling ball, or perhaps someone enjoying a few too many beers.

Dispatch told us we had a medical emergency, female patient, so our minds entertained thoughts of minor female complaints, not to worry. Of course, we both considered that some old retired person just dropped a gutter ball and then hit the floor with a massive MI, but we did not say it aloud. Karma, you know. Never think negative thoughts lest you draw them to yourself.

Arriving on the scene, we met with firefighters who had a less than in-control demeanor, not a good sign. We asked what we "had" inside (the nature of the call and complaint), and the firefighters shrugged their shoulders. We tried to get more information out of them, but they smirked a bit and said, "Naw, you gotta see this for yourselves." Bob and I looked at each other. He was amused, I took deep breaths.

Bob led the way with the gurney stacked high with our jump bag, Lifepak defibrillator, and portable oxygen (one never knows; remember the thoughts we keep to ourselves about possible codes). When we got into the area where the patient was resting, attended by discomfited firefighters, I walked over to her and took the lead, something I would never have done while working with Bob unless we had agreed beforehand who would attend.

This one was clearly mine; the stress fell away.

Admittedly, I stifled a giggle as I realized the reason the firefighters, normally exceptionally competent fellows, were so out of their element. The patient and the entire group around her were deaf, and hands were flying. The greater population of the bowling alley and everyone in this particular group were using sign language.

At the time, I communicated at about a third-grade level in American Sign Language: nothing to write home about, but enough to be able to communicate. The patient was most assuredly able to lip-read what I said to her, and write down questions and answers on paper if my limited sign language failed us. I knew this, but the other ES professionals around me did not.

Unfair advantage, you say? Score one for the girls.

I signed to the patient, "Hi, my name is Sherry, and I am here to help you. I do not sign much, so please sign slowly to me. What is wrong? What hurts?" The rest of the assessment was simple as the patient used small words and fingerspelled medications, more complicated thoughts, and any time my eyes crossed and glazed over in puzzlement. The patient was relieved that I had some appreciation for her situation, and I appreciated her patience with my limited ability to speak her language.

We delivered our patient to the ER, and I stayed with her, giving her paper and pen to communicate with the doctors and nurses. The nurse showed the same discomfort the firefighters had exhibited, and I apologized to the patient. She patted my hand as if to say, "I'm used to it," and it struck me that a woman in crisis was alone because the professionals' uneasiness was more important than the patient's needs. Those who feared they could not talk to her avoided her. I stayed with her until Bob finished cleaning the rig, and we moved on to our next call.

I often wondered if the twinkle in Bob's eye during this particular run was coming from a personal joke, a wandering thought, or if maybe old Bob was proud of his female partner and protégé. I never knew until we exchanged emails recently that the latter was true. Even though delayed, I can feel the inner satisfaction of making my partner, someone for whom I had such incredible respect, proud. Beyond the immeasurable satisfaction gained from taking good care of a patient, especially in challenging circumstances, the value of personal and professional recognition is incomparable.

Thanks, Bob. I love you, too.

~ ~ ~

Sometimes the day-to-day happenings are neither frightful nor delightful, but they paint an accurate picture of the things you may observe if you are paying attention. Often the little things in life amuse, bemuse, or infuriate us. How to perceive these items is entirely up to the individual. I would much rather find the humor and gifts in situations than concentrate on the negative energies of small minds. I may not always be successful, but I try.

Just Between Friends

One of my favorite groups of hospital residents (doctors in training) are the Family Practice folks. I never understood what made them so special, but they were always kind, considerate, took the best care of their patients, and treated ER RNs and staff courteously and with respect. It is no wonder that those folks were dearest to our hearts, and we could not do enough for them.

We fed them. We ran for coffee (sometimes the lousy ER stuff, but tired docs appreciate anything). We handed them half-smashed granola bars out of our book bags when we knew they'd failed to take time for breakfast or lunch. And even if we had acquired a chair only moments before (for the first time in 8 hours) we—well, I—often offered that seat, so the doc had a place to write orders. Family Practice (FP) docs gave patients bedpans, sometimes retrieving them after use, asking only where to deposit the contents and if the nurse needed a sample. What is not to love?

We took care of them when they were sick, too, although they rarely had to ask. Do you have a cough? Let me pull some Robitussin out of the drawer for you, and I think I have some Sudafed non-drowsy OTC (over the counter) in my bookbag. Uh, oh, is diarrhea problematic for you today? I know we have some Imodium in the drawer; I will get it for you *stat* (even though we never really said "stat").

Sometimes a pill and a prayer were not quite enough, and if the docs were bone-weary sick, they requested a shot, which is how Keith* and I became friends forever. You cannot help but become fast friends with a doctor who feels so miserable that he has no shame about lowering his drawers in front of you and bending over a patient gurney. I used the smallest gauge needle possible to deliver the medication. True to FP doc form, Keithie complimented my skills in painlessly administering the intramuscular (IM) injection.

It was our little secret, and I gave that shot without looking at the *target* (Keithie's bum). I felt for my physical landmarks, swabbed with alcohol, and shot between my fingers. Dr. Keith not only survived the illness and my injection, but also opened a practice, got married, had kids, and lived happily ever after. I never told him I did not look when I administered that shot.

Maybe I should drop him an e-mail and confess.

~ ~ ~

One of the rewards of being a medic or nurse in emergency medicine is the closeness we have with physicians. They are like family, and if we do not yet know them, an introduction through someone who does serves as permission to enter the inner sanctum. No one in ES ever wants to go to an ER as a patient. We know about the wait and the germs on the cot. We are aware of folks all around who are either throwing up on the floor while making horrendous retching sounds for emphasis, or coughing without covering to share their illness and prove they are sick.

As medics and nurses, we all too often come to work ill (not contagious) or in pain and sidle up to a friendly doc for some free advice. "Hey, doc—can you look at my throat (or other body part suffering illness or injury)?" The docs were quick to write a prescription, pull medication samples out of the resident's room left by drug reps, or refer us to the best specialist they knew if the problem was complex.

In the old days, we also had cooperative agreements with other departments. You take an x-ray of my thumb (that just jammed into the patient cot), and I will plug an IV into you with some meds for that nasty hangover. Do you need a breathing treatment for your asthma? No problem. As long as the doc orders it, let me pull this curtain around us, and away we go.

These days, medications and supplies are linked to a patient medical record number, as are tests such as x-rays. You cannot pull meds or perform a test without charging someone. Obvious legal and ethical issues prevent assigning these charges to patients, and there is only so much wiggle room for charging to "ER stock."

I miss the old days.

~ ~ ~

I left Detroit and my beloved trauma center several years ago, and until recently, I thought that door had closed. In May, I visited Michigan to see family and a few very close friends. One of those friends is Deb H., who has become a sister (of choice rather than blood), so we squeeze in a short visit when I am in town. Even though we are both graduate students battling fatigue and public drooling, one or both of us occasionally manages to make sense (usually Deb) before someone (usually me) zones out and has to be caffeine-resuscitated.

Deb is the interim manager of the ER that I called home for 11 years while another friend, Arlene, has moved temporarily to a different hospital (to reorganize the ER). Arlene and Deb met me at the door when I returned to those hallowed halls for the first time since leaving as an employee. This old Detroit ER nurse became a little *verklempt*. I felt like the returning prodigal son adorned with robes and greeted with open arms. I forgot to ask about the fatted calf.

The ER, completely transformed into one snappy operation, had features that years earlier we three could only imagine. There was a flat-screen TV in each room (enclosed by glass doors and private curtains), a computer terminal by each bed for bedside charting. There were tons of med stations, equipment and supplies, and all within reach of the patient care areas.

The best part was seeing old friends from when I'd started in the ER. One familiar and smiling face was that of Dr. Patricia N., an incredible ER physician and incomparable woman, who delivered glowing affirmations about my nursing skills. "You should come back; you are a really good nurse, and we need good nurses." Then she asked if she could hug me.

Deb led me away moments later because I started sobbing. I have been away from direct patient care for a year while writing and attending school, and somehow lost the sense that I still have value, that I am still a nurse. Just because I am not practicing right now does not mean I *used* to be a nurse or that I am a *retired* nurse. I *am* a paramedic, and I *am* a nurse, like my dad (who had not served in the military since Korea) never stopped being a Marine.

In Emergency Medicine, we all pay our dues as we immerse ourselves into one of the strongest families you may ever encounter. I saw Kathy B. that day, and Joe P., and Anita V., and Wendy S., and so many more. Even though I had not seen Dr. Doug W. in years, I walked over and kissed his cheek before even saying hello, and he responded in kind. The resident sitting next to Doug stared with an open mouth, and I may have said something inappropriate like, "I tend to wander into public establishments and kiss random men." We may not see one another for a very long time, but we are forever family. *Famiglia!*

My point is that if you see the staff in the ER or EMS services getting a little too chummy, or kidding around with great familiarity, or greeting one another with hugs and cheek-smoochies, it is ultimately in your best interest. People who genuinely care for one another and know each other well enough to demonstrate affection probably work very efficiently together, too. When the seams of civilization split, you want a crew that can work together efficiently, who have performed medical skills and procedures so many times they can almost do them blindfolded. Even though it may be *your* first experience, you do not want it to be theirs.

Trauma is not for sissies. For those of us who love trauma, who are addicted to it, who respond to it very well, this is our drug of choice. We are there for you, and even when we step away from our practice, we are still the professionals we were when we stood at your bedside. We are still Trauma Junkies. And by golly, I am still a darn good nurse.

~ ~ ~

If you work EMS in a small town, especially with a volunteer group, the ambulance company often waives the bill if you use their services. My young daughter had been ill with a fever that continued to rise in spite of all appropriate interventions, so she enjoyed a complimentary ride with Medic Jeff to the hospital. Her diagnosis was pneumonia, and the embarrassing moment of throwing up on Medic Jeff soon forgiven and graciously forgotten.

Not being the center of attention was difficult for Michele's father, Arnold,* who felt the need for attention and a free ambulance ride. Arnold had watched enough television to know the appendix was in the right lower part of the belly, so he called the ambulance complaining of acute right lower quadrant abdominal pain. A quick assessment showed no tenderness, no fever, no nausea or vomiting (signs of appendicitis), but Arnold insisted he was gravely ill.

Arnold did not pay as much attention to the TV shows as he should have. The classic presentation of abdominal pain includes doubling over in pain and guarding (protecting) the area that hurts. Instead, Arnold stiffened up like a board, threw his head back, locked his arms straight at his sides, and insisted he could not bend or walk.

The ambulance crew put the stretcher next to the couch to retrieve their patient as the crew and I exchanged glances. Jeff's partner did a little eye-rolling, and Medic Jeff's face had that, "You're taking me away from home for THIS?" look. I understood completely, shrugged, apologized, and told them if they wanted to dump Arnold on the side of the road, somewhere, anywhere, I would understand completely. I would be grateful.

Advice: if you are going to fake an illness, in this case, "pretend-icitis," please pay attention to the classic signs and symptoms, or you may become the butt of jokes and examples of "can you believe this?" conversations about ambulance calls. Seriously, even Ferris Bueller knew enough to hold his thermometer next to a light bulb to fake a fever.

~ ~ ~

On my way home from nursing school one afternoon, I saw our city EMS rig parked in front of a local liquor store. Because there were no fire vehicles (or personnel) present and I was a member of that EMS' volunteer corps, I decided to park my car, go inside, and see if my fellow EMTs needed assistance. Sometimes extra hands make life a lot easier, and we functioned as a team whether or not we were on duty. Because I was not wearing my pager, I had no idea what the folks were doing inside, or which crew was working.

When I went into the store, I saw an EMT holding a bag of IV fluid high in the air, and one of my regular partners, with a smirk on his face, taping down the IV tubing. The patient, pale and staring forward as though emotionally and mentally removed from the situation, was sitting up with a large, blood-soaked pressure bandage wrapped around his thigh. I asked the medic in charge if he needed anything, and he said, "Nope; got it covered, but thanks for stopping."

After the EMT loaded the patient into the rig for transport, I walked up to the medic and asked him to explain the smirk on his face. As he closed the ambulance doors, with his partner inside the ambulance attending to the patient, the smirk grew into a broad grin. The medic told me the patient had heard about people robbing liquor stores, so he purchased a gun in preparation for attempted robberies. The faithful employee wanted to be safe, protect his employer's assets, and quite possibly be a hero if anyone tried to rob him.

Fascinated with his new toy, the newbie firearm-owner took the gun and imagined scenarios calling for the use of deadly force, dodging bullets, and conquering bad guys. Unfortunately, the young man forgot the first rule of firearms: do not take a gun out unless you are prepared to use it. The inexperienced fellow was playing with a loaded gun, and (you guessed it!) delivered a self-inflicted gunshot wound to his leg. I guess he forgot about dodging friendly fire.

~ ~ ~

Let me preface the telling of this confession by saying it was not me. I do not have x-ray vision, nor would I dismiss a patient's complaint as unfounded, even if I considered it completely bogus. In EMS, we have "regulars," especially in extremes of weather, who want to get off the street. Hospitals are safe places that deliver tender loving care, "three hots and a cot" (food and shelter), brand spanking new hospital-quality footies with the rubberized non-skid safety strips on the bottoms, an occasional doctor-ordered foot cleansing including shaving cream soak, clean sheets, warm blankets, and all the requisite attention and service of a spa attendant (your nurse).

An old city EMS fellow left the rat race and came up to our sleepy town's relative calm and quiet (pardon the "Q" word, but I think we are safe while sharing stories). As a basic EMT working in an advanced (ALS) ambulance, this fellow liked to tell city stories to remind us that we were a bunch of newbies compared to him because he knew what *real* EMS was. I would not argue the point, but when you are at least 30 minutes from the nearest hospital, you become an ER on wheels and do more than load-and-go transports. That aside, we let Harry[*] ramble on about his experiences.

One of those stories was quite brief but stuck with me because it sounded more like urban legend than fact. Harry employed a technique for what he termed "BS Calls." I can appreciate not wanting to take an ambulance out of service for non-emergency situations, like a regular seeking free transport to the hospital, and seriously applaud the inventiveness of this particular maneuver. Again, no approval here, just acknowledging creativity and audacity.

Harry's ambulance had an x-ray machine. No, this is not a standard-issue item, and in larger cities, some may question the expenditure. No one but Harry and his partner knew of this special service, which was available in any rig that Harry worked (apparently, he took it with him). When Harry picked up the regulars who wanted a warm, free trip to the ER for complaints like, "I think I broke my leg" (the same leg the patient was walking on without difficulty the last two miles before realizing he was tired and wanted a ride), Harry employed his magic x-ray machine.

I could only imagine the procedure, but it reportedly worked every time. Harry had his partner (the driver) pull the rig into a darkened place between buildings, such as an alley (to gain maximum effect). Harry then dramatically positions the patient's extremity (whatever broke) and turned off all of the lights in the rig. The inside glowed with the auto-lights of buttons and radios so that Harry could see his patient well enough, and Harry's partner could watch for the signal.

Harry told the patient to hold his breath and signaled his partner in the front seat, who flashed the light bar on top of the rig, briefly echoing intermittent red flashes inside the patient compartment. Harry would then excuse himself and slip into the front compartment to wait for the x-ray to "develop." Soon Harry would return to the patient, reveal his findings (no break), have the patient sign off on the complaint (refused transport), and delivered the patient back to his starting point. Was it ethical or professional? Perhaps not, but you have to admit it was downright clever, and the kind of thing many of us in EMS secretly wish we could do.

~ ~ ~

In the business of patient care, especially in emergency services, you have about half a minute to establish a trusting relationship with patients before touching them in familiar ways (and private places). Emergency nurses do not have last names, for safety and security reasons. An exchange might go like this: "Hi, my name is Sherry, and I will be your nurse today. While the doctor asks you all sorts of questions that you may not consider pertinent, I am going to put holes in you where they did not exist before, and insert tubes in very uncomfortable places you wish I would not go. However, it's all part of giving you good care, so as much as it may hurt and embarrass you, because I am a total stranger, I am sure you will trust me completely to do what I understand to be right even if you do not." Something like that.

Accurately reading patients in those 30 seconds, and knowing how best to work with them is challenging. Beyond reading non-verbal communications is the conundrum of determining how to present explanations and care in a comforting, reassuring, professional, and natural way. Some people do not like nurses that kid around and smile, as those behaviors may be interpreted as uncaring considering the patient's pain (even when the complaint is minor).

Other folks get through their unexpected situation with humor, so reading the patient (especially the ones who may be dangerous), and communicating back to them appropriately, demands educated guesswork when the patient is stone-faced and stoic. Learning to read body language is a safety tool. It tells you how to deal with the patients and their families. ER folks quickly learn how to refine those skills.

I am usually good at reading people, but I have completely flopped too. My mind-reading skills malfunction if I forget to wear my cape and superhero shoes. Fortunately, after the initial 30 seconds of patient-professional bonding, kindness, genuine caring, and a warm smile go a long way. With many family-centered ethnic groups, a large group of concerned family members and friends participate in the patient treatment process, so trying to communicate effectively with all of them amid chaos sends you fishing for cues.

With one particular group, I was concentrating on a very difficult IV as the family spoke to one another and impatiently demanded answers before blood was drawn or tests completed. As I moved from one side of the bed to the other hanging IV bags and giving medications, I explained what I was doing. I also dealt with concerns and questions presented by family members who seemed to speak all at the same time, addressing the most important components first.

Suddenly, the whole family stopped talking.

They seemed oddly amused as they looked at one another, and the spokesperson of the group finally said, "You look European. Where are you from?" I said my family was from Moro D'Oro, Italy, but I was American born. The speaker cocked his head, squinted, and asked, "Your Mama or your Daddy is Italian?" I said Mama, and they all smiled.

Apparently, beyond my efforts to communicate with words and gestures was a non-verbal giveaway that caused them to relax, smile, and accept that their loved one would get the best care. My Italian nose and features conveyed more than I could with words, and for the duration of their crisis, I became a trusted part of the family. *La famiglia è tutto!* (Family is everything)

~ ~ ~

As a "Medic Du Jour," I rotated through various cars, shifts, stations, and partners. It was important for me to present exemplary work ethics, respect my partners and patients, and for the most part, bring Little Sherry Sunshine into the workplace to make each day easier. Eventually, most of the folks in the company accepted me. My reputation was of a "Girl Who Could Lift" in spite of being just a wee bit of a thing. It was not long before male partners adopted me as a little sister or because I was a seasoned veteran and over 35, a mom.

Part of the adoption process involved those partners showing me their tips for making life easier. EMS is all about improvisation and creative problem solving, and woe to those without common sense or critical thinking skills. Sometimes I learned things from the boys in situations when I did not realize there was a problem but accepted the creative solutions in anticipation of using them another time.

Bill* was a jovial fellow who told many jokes and worked smart, not hard. One of the tricks Bill shared was how to avoid potential dangers when picking up a patient in the ghetto deep into the night—without ever leaving the rig. Standard protocol demanded first going to the door and establishing the medical emergency, especially if the dispatcher sent us out to an "unknown" situation.

In ghetto neighborhoods, sometimes we left the driver in the rig, passenger door open, while the partner walked up to the patient's door. We never took equipment to the door in some inner-city neighborhoods because drug-seeking folks liked to call 911 for "chest pain," knowing the medics carried morphine. The partner who went to the door stood off to the side and knocked, knowing never to stand directly in front of the door lest greeted by gunfire. Bill had a better way, especially when he knew the address and the regular client who lived there.

We drove to a dark, run-down neighborhood that Bill knew well. Bill honked the horn, and the patient walked out, suitcase in hand, and let himself into the back of the rig. Bill told me to strap the fellow into the jump seat and take his vital signs sitting up. Getting a full report from Bill during the time it took the fellow to exit his front door and walk to the rig, I knew the complaint, medical history, medications, and allergies before the man sat down. All I had to do was fill in the report and check pulse, blood pressure, and respirations twice during the transport.

Neither Bill nor I minded having those easy calls, especially when it meant not having to do a major cleanup of the rig. Sometimes a break is a good thing, so instead of being annoyed at a "BS Call," Bill and I enjoyed the relative ease of a stress-free ride to the hospital. The lesson was to accept small gifts when you get them because you never know when the universe will grant another.

Then Bill showed me the coffee machine in a hospital waiting room that dispensed coffee without taking coins. Free hot chocolate and cappuccino was manna from Heaven, and par for Bill's contributions to my Street Smart Paramedic Continuing Education Program. Some of life's lessons are easy, and oh, so sweet.

~ ~ ~

OK, sometimes it is about drama and heartstring-pulling. These are the times when we feel useless, and wade through the mire of practicing protocols without getting caught up in emotion, especially if that emotion is personally threatening. If you throw cultural differences into the mix, with inherent misunderstandings, things can go downhill quickly. And when you thought you might walk away feeling rotten, someone says just the right thing to pull you back up into realizing that some things, like people dying, are not at all under our control.

Rule #1: People Die. Rule #2: Medics cannot change rule #1. (But boy, do we try!)

When Not to Work a Code

There are particular circumstances in EMS when someone in cardiopulmonary arrest will not receive the full bells and whistles treatment of Advanced Cardiac Life Support. If the patient no longer has a head, or if rigor mortis has set in, those are clear indications that CPR probably won't have successful outcomes. Under those circumstances, and others clearly outlined in EMS objectives and protocols provided by the states and agencies governing EMS workers, one does not work a code. However, there are times when it is unclear whether or not life-saving measures are appropriate.

My partner and I once responded to a home with a large family, celebrating some family tradition. To this day we are not completely sure what holiday it may have been, as most of the folks present did not speak English, but I maintain that it was simply Sunday dinner with a very close extended family. Dispatch informed us the patient was unresponsive, which usually indicates no pulse, no breathing, and drive fast, so we traveled lights and sirens a relatively short distance to a private home.

We were brusquely ushered into the living room of a large upscale home situated in a very expensive neighborhood. Upon entering the house, it took us a moment to locate our patient among the throngs. I estimated 73 people, and a quick look around the room assured that we had an audience paying particularly close attention to everything we did.

The patient was Grandma, lying supine on the couch with a scarf wrapped around her head. Grandma was looking quite pale and not breathing. Because there were three medics on the call that day, one fellow had the luxury of asking the family's spokesperson about Grandma's medical history. Most interestingly, he asked about the scarf wrapped from under Grandma's chin to a severe knot at the top of her head.

It seems Grandma was 103 years old, and at some point during the day, her jaw had dropped open and family, being helpful, wanted to close it, hence the scarf. In EMS, this represents a positive "O" sign, because the mouth forms a large letter "O," usually indicating a severe medical problem, like death. The family left Grandma to rest on the couch, with the scarf holding her jaw in a semi-closed position until they realized that Grandma had not moved in a very long time, and they could not remember the last time anyone saw her breathing. Of course, the situation became an emergency to the family at that point, but truthfully, Grandma had probably stopped breathing quite a long while before.

When faced with such a large number of family members, most of whom were talking loudly, crying, and pointing at Grandma with gestures we interpreted as, "Do Something Now," one tends to the job at hand without ceremony. We hooked the patient up to the cardiac monitor (no rhythm) and attempted an IV in the patient's foot (no other veins). CPR was active at this time, and the patient was a bit stiff, indicating that she had probably died a few hours before. Our highly developed intuitive senses tingled at the thought of doing anything less than a full code ("Danger, Will Robinson!").

In spite of Grandma having reached well past the century mark, the family was not ready to let her go. The fear and pain in their eyes, the sense of urgency in the room, the panicked movements of everyone who felt so utterly helpless washed over us like an emotional wave. We knew we had to give the family something to hang onto, something they could tell the rest of the family: *the EMS Paramedics and the doctors and nurses at the hospital did everything they could to save Grandma, but she was gone. It was God's/Allah's/The Universe's will.* My heart ached a bit for all of them as the unthinkable happened before their eyes. Goosebumps rose on my arms, a subtle indication, even though I remained without facial expression, that this call affected me personally. I would address those feelings later, after the call.

Blood had not been moving through Grandma's veins for a while, so the IV fluid was not flowing. I taped the catheter to her foot to expedite moving her out to the ambulance and continuing the show. I was in the vein, but the vein was not pushing blood, even with more than adequate cardiac compressions.

My partner was unable to open the locked jaw, so intubation was out of the question. A bag valve mask pushed air. We secured the patient onto the backboard and then the stretcher, and quickly moved into the ambulance and on to the hospital. We continued ACLS (Advanced Cardiac Life Support) procedures throughout the transport.

My grandmother died during a personally trying time in my life as I juggled divorce, full-time nursing school, three jobs, and 800 miles a week travel. I rarely slept more than three hours a night and was exhausted. Before Gram died, I secretly considered quitting nursing school, but when I saw Gram to say goodbye, I slipped my student ID into the casket and promised that I would see my education through. I graduated with high honors and four degrees in two years. I empathized with that family, knowing Grandmothers are sometimes the glue that holds a family together.

It may have seemed medically bizarre to work a code on a 103-year-old patient who had been dead for a while, but it made sense emotionally. We were not offering anyone false hope; we were showing them that we humans can do everything right and sometimes the outcome is far beyond our reach. Their faith and their family would keep them strong, bind them closer, and they could celebrate a life filled with love in their way.

The hospital staff prepared for us, as we had radioed in ahead of time with a full report, repeating the patient's age twice. The doctor knew from our descriptions and interventions that he would probably "call" (end) the code shortly after we arrived, and he did. Still, a little good-natured ribbing was in order, and the ER doctor's first question, as we moved the patient from our gurney to his, was, "Really? You worked this one. Must we have that conversation again about when NOT to work a code?"

We could tell by the twinkle in his eye and amused look that he KNEW we had a good reason for initiating care. His demeanor helped to turn a bad situation into one about which we were all proud. Those who did not understand our efforts, who belabored the paperwork and effort we "caused" them, missed the point. I can only hope they understand before they have to view it from the other side of the gurney.

POSTMORTEM

The retrospection following an earlier chapter touched on gallows humor, something about which I was aware since first starting in EMS. I know civilians didn't understand it, and I peeked around corners with my peers before sharing stories lest someone heard us. I knew back then that some people got completely burned out and left, often at the end of a workweek, sometimes in the middle of a shift. What I did not understand the first decade or two was how some people could laugh and be seemingly untouched by what they experienced, and others melted into a puddle.

So I did some research. Well, a lot of research. Graduate school was a foray into crisis management and response (MS Psychology). The doctoral journey allowed perusal into what fascinated me the most: the effects our careers have on us emotionally, personally, and professionally, and what we can do about it. Secret: I titled my doctoral dissertation with an acronym, so I could remember it (medical trick). NOTERaCE. Nurses' Occupational Trauma Exposure, Resilience, and Coping Education. If interested, you may download the dissertation (for free) at https://scholarworks.waldenu.edu/dissertations/2360/.

The short version is that high levels of occupational exposure to traumatic stress, combined with few opportunities for resilience and coping training, contribute to disengagement, crises of competence, and burnout. Some of us, exposed to trauma after trauma, and without training in coping and resilience, pull away, feel we cannot do the job, and become exhausted in the effort to continue paddling at the deep end of the pool. We. Are. Toast.

Conversely, some folks experience compassion satisfaction, which is a positive feeling of accomplishment following delivering patient care, even if the outcome was not what might have been desired or anticipated. Sometimes, satisfaction from professional identification, academic accomplishments, and clinical competencies intrinsically and outwardly enmeshed in the meaning attached to professional roles outweigh negative outcomes. The patient died, but we expertly did everything we could, and nothing we might have done additionally or differently would have changed the outcome. We feel elated, more than competent, dropping a few coins in the jar of our purpose and meaning, and we head home.

Something else we may do, on the way home, is an intentional act to transition between what some call "Hell and home." Some folks have rituals; I mentioned taking a deep breath and blowing out to the horizon of the lake as I drove home. Others tap parts of their car interior while lifting their feet off the floor driving over the same railroad tracks they cross going to and from work. Others may have a piece of clothing or equipment that goes on and off to signify working/off work. The point is to live a life of intention, of control, of separation so that we are not our jobs; we are not completely defined by them. They are parts, not the whole.

Part V

Crisis and Disaster Response

No matter how long I have been in crisis response, that very first call still gives me pause. The truth is that I do not want to receive those calls. They mean that folks are hurting because of a tragedy somewhere. Little Sherry Sunshine wants happiness, peace, and love the world over, no nicks, cuts, bruises, fractured bones, and please, please, please no broken hearts!

Underneath the Detroit Medic/RN, tough-guy exterior is a four-year-old girl enmeshed in eternal hope, a girl who once brought a dead dog home and put it in Mama's bed for healing. If there has to be pain in this world, there has to be healing. That hope is what motivates this ER Chick to continue to try to make things better. In crisis management and response, that first notification, and first step toward healing, usually comes via telephone.

Getting the Call

I came home from a 12-hour ER shift, kicked my shoes off at the door, and jumped into the shower to wash off the drudgery and pathologic exposures accumulated through a very busy and demanding day. Once cleansed of stressors and germs, all washed unceremoniously down the drain with a sigh of relief, I sat down at my desk to tackle a second full-time job as a national para-military crisis response team-leader, trainer, and interventionist. When my fatigued brain recognized the red blinking light of the answering machine, I listened to an emotionally affected leader, relaying a tragedy within his ranks.

Our emergency services and disaster response workers expected natural disasters, like floods and hurricane damage, or even airplanes falling out of the sky. In every training, folks were cautioned that sometimes the worst thing that could happen in a search and rescue operation was that they would find what they were looking for; what then? We discussed at length how to respond to the blood, guts, and emotional gore involved in disaster relief and crisis response, but this call was different.

Reflecting the culture and human-made tragedies of the day, when guns and people encounter one another without respect to person or age, this call was about an adolescent shot in the head. It would be wonderful to say that I snapped into work mode and immediately began to rally the crisis response team, but I did not. This was my first major incident, and gaining composure took a few minutes.

I put my head down on my desk and felt a wave of nausea pass through me like a corrosive mist. My head was swimming with the realization that these folks expected me to know what to do, to help them, a responsibility that weighed heavily demanding every available ounce of energy and effort. Then, I took a few deep breaths, replayed the message, writing pertinent facts on the CISM Team Request Form, and prepared myself for returning the Commander's call.

The Commander was heartsick. The accident did not occur during a mission or have any connection to our formal organization, but the person shot was well known, and the urgency of the situation magnified by the age of the victim. The incident was several states away, so we relied on local volunteer CISM agencies to supplement our peer and professional staff for the planned psychological first aid intervention (ICISF Model Debriefing). Preparations for a structured group discussion began on the next assigned meeting night at the regular meeting place. With appropriate contacts made, permissions gained, and intervention funding approved, I flew south to meet with the folks.

We expected 20 people, 27 arrived, and those who were in management roles said they understood if they could not participate in a formal debriefing. The leaders knew because of their training that we shied away from mixing groups of command staff and worker bees. The two PsyDs and I discussed how to handle this group, deciding that splitting them into subgroups could be detrimental.

The folks present had equal experience and exposure to the crisis. Meeting together would reinforce their strengths and cohesiveness. We had assessed the group in a pre-meeting informal gathering, touched by their unselfish and unswerving dedication to each other, the organization, and, most importantly, by the leaders toward the people in their charge.

The folks made our jobs easy as we led them through the formality of a debriefing, allowing them to share, educating them, providing resources, and letting them know we were available after the debriefing. During the meeting and informal gathering afterward, "milk and cookie time," we four crisis team responders (two MHP PsyDs and two peers) had an after-action support meeting with one another. Assured that the debriefers suffered no ill effects from the intervention, we bid goodbye to the local troops and went our separate ways.

This crisis response was my first "big one" and I admit to post-intervention emotional exhaustion. I could see how people who did this type of work for extended periods burned out. Kevin, the pilot who flew me back home to Michigan, asked several questions during the flight, which I did not hear. Kevin finally put his hand on my arm and asked if I was OK, bringing me back to the inside of the plane instead of inside my head.

I had not heard a single word, but felt like the Incredible Hulk shrinking back into Dr. David Banner, replete with tattered emotional remnants, the effects of functioning at full-tilt until the emergency passed. The mission was complete and successful. All of the incredible stress and strain of the preceding days gathering people and making arrangements was over, and I could rest. I crashed.

Eventually, learning how to be empathetic without losing myself in the process took discipline, education, and training. My cautionary statement to all in crisis management and response is not only self-care but also self-awareness. Support systems are unquestionably important. Use them, get feedback. Reality checks are also important for survival. If you use all of your fuel without replenishing, the engine eventually stops, and you are dead on the road.

Refuel, renew, use your supports, and please take care of yourself. You never know when the phone will ring, and you want to be prepared to take that very important call.

Neophytes in crisis management take many classes in various models of crisis intervention. My experiences and preferences the past few decades have been to embrace ICISF (International Critical Incident Stress Foundation) Model, as an interventionist, an ICISF Approved Instructor, and now as ICISF Faculty. Some of the things I have learned, observed, and practiced may be of interest. Those memoirs follow.

The Teacher is In ...

Maj Wendy, MSW, was interviewing potential instructors for her USAF CISM training. She asked if my classes were boring, and I replied, "Of course they are boring: there's a lot of mental health stuff!" Wendy once attended a CISM course where the instructor wrote every word of the two-day lecture on a flip chart. Wendy later told me that comparatively, my course was like Disneyland and I am optimistically keeping that review in memory as a compliment.

Students can expect to learn, to prepare for what is out there, and to function independently without Mama Sherry. I have so much to learn, but I have been told by the pros that my instincts are "110% correct," so I trust them. As a graduate student in psychology (specializing in crisis management and response), I am finding that education exponentially enhances experience and instinct. This section is an effort in sharing what happens when an ES Trauma Junkie becomes a crisis intervention helper.

Everyone has different methods of teaching and learning. CISM course participants often represent diverse educations and professions, especially with volunteer groups. My course locations range from sparse Army camps to luxury hotels, as arranged by the course requestors. Attendees occupationally and educationally range from mechanics to medical doctors, high-school graduates to PhDs, and MHPs to those seeking solutions for personal mental health issues. With mixed groups, classes physically divide into like-minded pockets of ES, cops, mental health, paramilitary, chaplains, and so on.

Part of teaching CISM courses involves breakout sessions after reviewing housekeeping items and making introductions. The kids get to play, and by this time in every class, my shoes are tossed aside, I have lost a solid 4" in height, and I no longer stand anywhere near the podium. I give students folded post-it notes with words on them, the students line up on either side of the classroom, and individually stand front and center to pantomime their assignments. Happy, sad, mad, bored, closed-minded, cold, not paying attention, surprised, impatient, ready to punch somebody, and desperately having to pee (my favorite) find expression through gestures. Blood circulates, brains refresh, and participants bond, more invested in the success of the classroom experience.

Moving on to verbal sharing (they have already introduced themselves, which is historical information, factual and safe), thoughts and opinions, and sometimes personal revelations and storytelling, opens folks up further and prepare them to experience feelings. The class becomes a reflection of crisis response intervention itself as we methodically travel from facts to thoughts to feelings.

Storytelling is important, as complex concepts break through the palpable fog of theory. By the time the class practices an actual group crisis intervention, students are ready to get into character and participate fully. Sometimes folks are so into their role-playing, desiring to portray accurately the emotions one might expect in particular circumstances, that they get into a place inside themselves that is hard to escape from. Other times they are just darn good actors, and fellow students practice discernment in differentiating between the two.

Let me describe for you one classroom experience when the participant was *not* acting.

I provided the background story and scenario ahead of time, so folks were familiar with the next day's breakout session. As we began, the group sat in chairs arranged in the traditional circle configuration, and each had a character assignment. Actors were playing either ES workers who responded to the crisis, or they were part of the crisis response team helping the ES folks. The two groups gathered separately for a moment and prepared their plan of action.

We had discussed appropriate and inappropriate touching, when to pay attention to a person, when to provide silent support, and advisements such as why we do not yell, "Oh My God Are You All Right," if someone is crying. During the CISM debriefing demonstration I stayed outside the group, as I had an experienced MHP in the class who needed to practice leading a debriefing (not counseling), and we had a painfully small class. Things seemed to be going well, until the person acting as the paramedic for the scenario became tearful, stood up, and walked out of the room.

My instincts sensed more than acting, so I followed. The woman threw her arms around my neck, weeping from a long-ago wound that opened during the breakout session. She was not ready to talk. I held on and held her up, allowing her to begin addressing the pain of something so gut-wrenching that she was using a total stranger as a life raft. And that's what happens in class, and in real interventions. Old wounds tear open because the superficial and inadequate bandage placed on them eventually wears away, often at the most incomprehensible and unexpected moments.

This woman was a strong, independent professional who had pulled herself up by her bootstraps more than once, starting over and building again after personal losses. Like most folks, her Achilles heel was children. She had an experience so personal and painful that she had kept it to herself, never truly mourning, never addressing the details lest they cause a complete collapse of her emotional house of cards built on sandy soil.

As a volunteer ES worker in real life, she had lost a child, a beautiful, sweet, innocent soul who loved popsicles, gave kisses to anyone who presented a cheek and giggled at birds and butterflies. The circumstances were unexpected and random, and the woman slowly deteriorated from the inside out as she assumed responsibility for something that was not her fault. Blame needed a place to land, and looking at the universe, or fate, or ultimately God as a cause made no sense, so she blamed herself. In an unprotected moment, pretending about a scenario that was not real, her protective walls came tumbling down, and she feared to drown in the flood of emotions that poured over her.

Eventually, the student portraying the crisis team interventionist in the doorkeeper role realized she was supposed to follow the woman who'd left the room. The doorkeeper bounced into the area where we stood, where I was holding a weeping woman up lest the weight of her memories caused complete collapse. The doorkeeper smiled broadly. "Hey! I thought we weren't supposed to hug!"

You know that "mom-look" that says leave now or (insert appropriate threat here)? I must have had that look on my face because I only had to whisper, "Go," and the doorkeeper went back behind the closed door into the room with the others who were still practicing. We talked later, and the doorkeeper understood that this had been a real situation.

Back together with the class, we discussed how sometimes even the CISM team members could lose their footing when a large wave comes in threatening to sweep them under. We talked about how in every debriefing, every intervention, there is an expected unexpected moment. If you anticipate that moment, and then recognize it, you are more prepared to deal with it. Those moments become "Aha, here it is, I can handle this" rather than "OMG, what the heck do I do now?"

The woman who had relived a past tragedy found a way to discuss her situation with someone appropriate that day. We had a slew of chaplains in camp, many of whom were mental health professionals. The chaplain stayed in touch with the woman as long as necessary, and I followed up with her for many months afterward. We discussed what happened during class and healthy ways to deal with stress. On the positive side of the fence, she wanted to learn more.

Folks I have met through the years, especially those who have had a particularly disturbing experience or see me as a newfound best friend, stay in touch for a time. I know they are doing well not only by the content of their communications but the frequency. When the communications slow and drop off, we have completed our journey together.

As a nurse, I give shots, pills, and treatments; I apply salves to some wounds, wrapping others with bandages and splints. I teach folks the road to physical healing using every trick I have accumulated through the years. However, we are more than our physical being; we also have minds and spirits. If we do not treat those three things as a complete entity, then we are doing a disservice to those with whom we professionally interact.

Recognizing the ill-effects of acute and chronic stress on our emergency services folks is paramount to their survival.

Remembering the classes I have taught, the people who have that "Aha!" moment as it all comes together and makes sense to them, is extremely rewarding. Hearing the stories from those students who go out and do great things, those who embrace the positive and help others to reframe experiences contribute to the logic of my existence. I am so very proud of them all.

I also remember those who faced their demons in an unexpected time and place, who held on with a white-knuckled death-grip. I remember the days some of them accepted that they were not so tough after all, and being human was not a bad thing. I remember them and pray for them, and hope they are doing well.

~ ~ ~

Hurricane Katrina devastated the Gulf Coast of Mississippi in September of 2005. As a team leader, my task involved developing and implementing a crisis response plan for paramilitary emergency services workers. Even though many of the workers' experiences were positive, some feelings stirred by prior familiarity with threatening or disaster events loomed, ready to spill emotional goo over everyone. This story includes the revelations of one ES responder during and after his defusing, personal and painful memories carried by a soldier who'd served in Vietnam. His contributions to this story provide the history beneath his unexpected reactions in a post-Katrina crisis intervention.

Post-Katrina: A (Military) Responder's Recollection

In crisis response, one learns rather quickly that we are not dealing exclusively with the obvious or expected, even following a clearly defined disaster. When our crisis response team met in Jackson, MS, to provide Critical Incident Stress Management (CISM) services to paramilitary responders, we anticipated encountering a grief and loss situation because of the utter devastation. What we found were dedicated volunteer groundpounders and aircrews, frustrated because they wanted to deploy much earlier, disappointed because they felt they hadn't done enough. Because of these two points of contention, many troops felt disheartened; they hadn't completed completed the mission to their satisfaction.

The workers learned those frustrations were not unusual, or specific to Katrina, but a common theme with rescuers from other major disasters. ES workers voicing similar dissatisfactions during CISM defusings helped dispel the fallacy of uniqueness, and some frustrations fell away, permitting reframing the work in a more positive light. Research tells us that positive support postcrisis exposure goes a long way toward mediating negative emotional experiences and pathological sequelae. We attempted to provide support and education during the intervention, and after the troops returned home.

Emergency service folks responding to disaster bring with them individual histories and experiences, including their methods of coping, ethics, perceptions, and perspectives. We need to be aware that any or all of these particulars may jump into the middle of a moment that we thought was about something else, the proverbial shoe one expects to drop at the most inopportune time. As with any disaster response plan, strategies can look great on paper but may hit the circular file during actual missions. Often the first item discarded in disaster response is Plan A. We regroup, reformulate, and design Plan B, sometimes as firm as Jell-O made with swamp water and just as tasty. Semper Gumby and rigid flexibility are the rule rather than the exception.

This story shares some details from an emergency services worker's perspective and history, including how his response to crisis intervention threw Plans B and C out of the window. Bob* is a paramilitary ground pounder who served as an active military troop in Vietnam, carrying his war-altered worldview through every aspect of his life. Far too complex for this book, PTSD is one of those issues that may surface in a post-event crisis team response. Often triggered by the similarities between the disaster and remembered war scenes, or by triggers seen by the ES worker that we may not comprehend, PTSD can be part of anyone's personal history.

Bob proudly wore a Civil Air Patrol (CAP) cadet uniform in an era when adolescents mocked and bullied contemporaries who wore military-type clothing. The public was less than supportive of military service. In 1968, Bob continued that military path by joining the Army.

"I wanted to do my part in the military. When I enlisted, I went to Fort Campbell (KY) for basic training, [then] airborne training, and from there to Special Forces training… it was pure hell. [We learned] how to disarm mines and how to kill your enemy quietly and swiftly. We had POW training at Fort Polk [using] a mock POW camp. It was 130 degrees inside during the day. Our mission was to kill people in Vietnam and recon, to gather all the intel we could. We would work behind enemy lines in Cambodia [and] Laos."

His descriptions of the training are brutal and disturbing. Bob adds that he cross-trained in weapons, demolition, and flying Huey helicopters. That training and experience provided enormous trigger potentials for his later participation in disaster relief operations held in an area hot, humid, and decimated like a war zone. Bob adds, "I was proud to be the best and be in Vietnam. When I came home, people at the airport would spit on me and call me a baby killer, [telling me] how wrong I was for killing those innocent people."

Trying to put negative experiences behind him, Bob saw his involvement with a paramilitary organization designed to help people as another way to serve proudly in uniform. He wanted to meet and exceed expectations of duty assignments, to share the helpful things he had learned.

"Maybe I could train young people how to survive in all kinds of weather and terrain, in the woods, how to find your directions if lost, to use a compass and give location by a grid on a map. [I wanted to teach] how to make litters and care for victims, how to make a shelter with nothing but what you can find in the woods, how to keep from freezing if you are stuck outdoors, and how to treat and know heat exhaustion. I am a disabled Vet, wounded two different times. [By teaching others] how to save lives instead of taking lives, I thought I could get some of my soul back and feel better about myself [and to regain] peace of mind."

Katrina promised, in Bob's view, a way to meet expectations of making a positive difference, maybe healing old wounds. Before the Katrina troops released from duty to head home, the mission SOPs (standard operating procedures) included mandated outbriefings (a term designed to cover all appropriate CISM interventions). Members from FOBs (forward operating bases) stopped at the mission headquarters (HQ), and attended group discussions led by Joan, a PsyD certified in thanatology (death, grief, and loss), and me.

Our HQ provided shelter, offices for operations, and an airplane hangar serving both air and ground crews during and after their sorties (individual maneuvers). We were grateful for the roof over our heads and running water. We met in an office turned bunking area for defusings. It was hot but private, and adequate to meet with each ground team and aircrew.

Joan and I had performed multiple defusings in addition to other minor Ops duties between interventions. I was in the uniform of the day, BDUs (battle dress uniform) that contained several patches identifying me as a peer to the ES folks. We discovered workers were more receptive to us if one of the CISM team members had similar background, training, and experience as the ES workers, a silent chisel effectively chipping away at their protective trauma armor.

Normally, I turned my collar upside down for interventions, hiding the Lt Col rank, but for this group, a little voice told me to leave the collar alone. Joan, my former student in CISM courses, reminded me of my teaching to hide the rank, but I smiled and said, "Not this time." Displaying rank was unusual, but some knowledgeable MHPs told me always to follow my gut instincts, so I did.

We formed a makeshift circle for our meeting, sitting on cots or the floor. When the group came into the room, they found Joan and me positioned across from one another in the circle, and Bob sat on the cot next to me. During our structured discussion, Bob had a particularly strong reaction, seemingly incongruent with the situation and topic, aimed at authority figures, particularly officers.

Bob turned to face me, loudly expressing feelings about officers who don't know what they are doing. He listed frustrations, like officers who lead troops blindly, who lack intelligence and integrity, who do not give a rat's [behind] about anyone but themselves. Bob complained about officers not only experience-deficient but those who sit at desks making bad decisions. The size 10 boot dropped squarely into my lap.

Bob was red-faced and angry, nose to nose with me and about an inch from my face. The room was silent. Trauma nurse instincts told me I was not in danger, that Bob had just cracked open a door and dared me to walk through.

Without blinking or backing away, I removed my overblouse, displaying the same uniform Bob wore: a brown t-shirt, BDU pants, and black boots. I said, "There is no rank in this room. We are equals. I appreciate you sharing how you feel, but let me make one thing very clear: I am here for you. I am here for YOU, Sarge. At this moment, it's just you and me in this room, and I am here for you."

The strangest thing happened after what my PsyD Joan later described as a "ballsy move." Bob backed away, grinned, and sat quietly for the rest of the discussion, contributing appropriately. I didn't know why or if what I said was the right thing to say; perhaps it was a very dumb thing to say, but my heart said it honestly, and it seemed to be what Bob needed to hear.

As promised, members of the crisis response team followed up with the folks we had talked to, mostly by phone, because of the geographical distribution of troops. Bob was mine. I talked to him on the phone and via email, finally learning that he had far more on his plate than Katrina, including a diagnosis of PTSD (Vietnam) and ongoing counseling. What this story reveals came well after the fact of the mission and defusing. I knew nothing about Bob or his history until long after the Katrina mission closed, and we returned home. Bob shared his expectations of Katrina and what happened during the defusing in an email to me.

"When I found out we were going to help people in Mississippi, I thought, and now I can save lives and not take them. When it was all over, I met you. We were in the room for [outbriefing] before we could go home, and in you came. There were about 8 of us. Everyone kept looking at me to start this off. I remember you saying Sarge, do you want to state anything?"

"I was PI—ED OFF because I felt that [I was kept] from doing my job, saving lives. I felt like I didn't accomplish my mission. Sure, we gave out food and water, but we didn't go where we were needed: Biloxi. I told [my major] that I was going to give them food, they needed food, [but] we were told to stay out of there because they were shooting people in uniform."

"When I was talking to you, I got a feeling that I have known you all my life. I could feel what was in your heart that you really cared what happens to us and everyone. When I was sitting on the bed, I wanted to get up and tell you I was sorry for being angry at myself for not doing my job. I guess I knew that I would see you again. You being a [Lt Col] and me a sergeant, I thought I better shut up before I got into trouble. Sergeants have a big mouth [and] mine gets into trouble all the time."

"I thank God for bringing us close together that day In Mississippi. I will always be there for you if you need me. I guess I could feel the hurt that you had inside of you the same as I do. In a way, I wanted to take all your hurt out of you and put it into myself."

Ever the soldier and protector, Sergeant Bob wants to keep the rest of the world safe, an impossible mission because of the realities of wars in and outside our shores. He will not give up, nor will any of us in crisis intervention or emergency services, the hats many of us wear on any given day, because we have hope that we can make a difference and keep the Boogeyman at bay. Sometimes we have positive outcomes, and sometimes, *sometimes,* we win. Finding ways to resolve past hurts is not part of the formula in psychological first aid, but knowing what some responders bring with them accentuates the importance of appropriate post-incident psychological aftercare.

Bob told me of "many nights that I sit and cry because I hurt inside and think of the friends I have lost in Vietnam. I wonder why I made it, and they got killed. The pain that I have inside me will never be able to get out.

"Many times, I wish I would [have] got out of this world. I have done many things for my country that I cannot talk about, and I have seen a lot of soldiers die for our country for you to give you freedom." Seeing Bob's phrase "*for you* to give you freedom" reminded me of what I'd said to him during the defusing: "*For you. I am here FOR YOU.*"

Bob later shared part of his journal: "When I met Sherry, it was our outbriefing, and I was really going to give them a piece of my mind. [Seeing that Sherry was a Lt Col], there was no way I could say what I wanted to say out of respect of her and her rank. I told her that, and she took off her uniform blouse and said there is no rank. That really stunned me. Later on I kept in touch with her by email. It was like a bond between us and I just adopted her as my little sister. I talk to Sherry because I trust her and I know that my little sister would not steer me wrong. She has made me see a lot of things in a different way. In a way I owe her my life. I have thought about getting out of this world, and when I feel that way I turn to Sherry. I don't tell her that, but just talking to me really helps."

I am not a mental health professional, but trust that I know when to contact them. I am a graduate student in psychology, specializing in crisis management and response. We do not counsel in CISM, but peer crisis responders must realize the tremendous responsibility involved in crisis intervention. Bob shared his innermost feelings in this book so that others might understand the gravity and necessity of crisis intervention following emergency services operations.

Bob adds a final thought: "Sis, if it wasn't for talking to you and the emails, I would have probably checked out of life." That sentence is significant in so many ways. Crisis intervention is tough work, certainly not for sissies, but the victories make sloshing around in the mud or debris while hungry, hot/cold, and far from home is incredibly rewarding. You cannot put a price on a life, or a friend, and Katrina gave me the immeasurable and unexpected gifts of both.

POSTMORTEM

When the last "anniversary" of our Joint Task Force (JTF) Katrina service rolled around, social media provided a private back room where we could meet, out of the public eye, and reminisce. The heaviness we'd brought home with us then, the change in worldview, has molded into a tightly-knit group of folks now who celebrate our unity, our friendship, our lifelong tie, embracing the purpose that led us to serve in the first place.

We pop into that private chat group on occasion when something from Katrina, or 911 (some of our folks served there, too), jogs our memories. "Hey guys, I'm just thinking about y'all today on this 9/11. I tell people sometimes that I have two different 9/11 memories, one good and one bad. Y'all are part of the good one. I hope y'all are well." Another posted a meme of a prayer that held him up and shared it to buoy us. Our ideologies differ wildly, yet are not divisively part of this familial equation.

Owen Y., Russ M., Eric H. ("Hud"), Ricky O. We are emergency services trained yet from different civilian professions. Most are pilots and command staff on the paramilitary/military side, who occasionally share pictures from the air that might include hints of the latest disaster or threat.

Outside this central core are more of those who served with us and continue the Katrina relationships. I get texts from one former cop, Paul B., "PrayN4U," who always seem to come when I need them most. Pastor Don B. is my Texas spiritual advisor, and Don and Paul are serious Prayer Warriors. Auntie Joan, the PsyD with me at Katrina HQ, has since dubbed me

"Aunt Sherry," a compliment and invitation to sit with her at the mental health folks' big kids table. Bob, the Viet Nam veteran who had a profound experience in the Katrina story, sends emails when the mood strikes. He calls me his little sister, tells me how he is doing, and if the weather has been favorable for riding his motorcycle. This past week, Bob joked that he recently had a total knee replacement because "the doctor said jumping out of airplanes (in the war) wears a joint out."

We held each other up; we hold each other up. The continuity between then and now is that time has not lessened our bond.

We peek in and wish each other well, catch up on a few details of life, and move on. Sometimes those wishes include mention of folks who have died, and we wonder if they are watching from a point we cannot see. One of the group suggested a reunion; we are planning for next year, outside of hurricane season, in a location that brings together folks from Texas to Michigan and up the east coast. Hud tells Owen he should fly out and pick us up, even though chartering a jet is unrealistic. One thing is sure: won't be a dry eye in the place.

(In Memoriam, Brigadier General Rex E. Glasgow, CAP)

POST-POSTMORTEM

We change over time. We soften or harden, become more understanding or cynical, gain great insight, or retreat into a cave of darkness. Our lives, our hearts, our minds, our psyches, our souls, one continuous Choose Your Own Adventure Series—marked by events that produce scars we proudly display or disguise and deny. Those in emergency services, military, paramilitary, medicine, nursing, PD, FD, EMS... we make choices every day, with every incident that leads to the next step, the next direction.

Earlier I mentioned highly sensitive people, people who ooze empathy, as well as those who have built effective trauma armor to protect themselves. Sometimes the same person can toggle between the two. Looking back, those prepared for impact had a better chance of surviving with minor scratches, and those who had strong support systems came through even when completely blindsided. I'm an Empath, an HSP, and have learned over the years how to protect myself. A Reiki Master friend, who expresses concern over my trials by fire, says I need to ground myself, to place a protective bubble around me. I tell her that I am a bubble master.

I am privileged to know some people who display amazing strength, who have hearts of gold, are empathetic, yet can walk over coals and heal from those burns. Asking them how they got through assures me that they are OK, and informs of what coping mechanisms they have developed to demonstrate such resiliency.

One such friend, whom I have adopted as an ED little sister, lives in Las Vegas. She worked with an ER doctor I know, and have known since he was a pup (ER resident) in Detroit, MI. Their particular experience pulls at my heartstrings.

You may have heard or read about a shooter opening fire on concertgoers at the route 91 music festival on the Las Vegas strip, killing 58 and wounding 413. The shooter fired more than 1100 rounds before turning the gun on himself (he shall not be named here out of respect for those affected by this tragedy). The ER RN, Debbie B., shares some of her thoughts and feelings about the shooting. She writes:

> I remember saying to my husband Saturday night, September 30, 2017, "We should try and go to the Route 91 Harvest Festival next year."
>
> "Sounds great," he replied.
>
> Fast forward 24 hours. I am getting ready for my shift. Talking with my favorite doctor about a rash on my hand (a rash he diagnosed as "goat clap" since I live on a farm, which the doc references in his presentations about that night), quickly turned into the worst night of my life.
>
> "Mass casualty, multiple shooters, county music concert." Those words rang out loud and clear!
>
> I promise you, no amount of E-learnings or Health-stream assignments can prepare you for those words. I ran on autopilot the whole night, except for just TWO moments! Firstly, the 10-minute wait in the ambulance driveway anticipating the worst and hoping for the best. Secondly, when I was told to stop doing CPR on a very

young girl who was already deceased when she got to me. Other than that, it was just go, go, go.

But we got through it. We made it. We had one of the doctors checking on us constantly. I did interviews and stories and talks. I tried to share my experience. The main thing I wanted to share:

NO MATTER WHAT, YOU ARE NEVER PREPARED!!

Before my involvement in the medical aftermath of this mass casualty shooting, I looked at events in the world and felt bad, but knew nothing like that would ever happen to me or anyone I love. That stuff doesn't happen where I am.

Now I go to events and search for all the emergency exits right away. I can walk into any venue and tell you exactly how many ways out there are. I watch people very carefully now. Watch their mannerisms. Watch what kind of baggage they are carrying. Look around at all the passengers on a plane.

I set up emergency plans with my family. When we are at a huge outdoor event, I set up meeting places should we become separated in a crisis. I also let them know I will be heading to any medical tent or hospital because that's just what I do. I do not let myself have a good time. But I also do not take those good times for granted any longer.

My family has been beyond supportive. They sat silently at first, waiting for me to talk about what I had witnessed and what I had done that night. The main doctor that night who I was side by side with pulling bodies out of cars has been more than supportive. All the medics that were dropping off patients to us that night— we all share a special bond. This incident has become a part of my life now. 10/1/17 was not just a "rough night at work." It made an impression that I can never erase. And, quite frankly, I honestly do not think I would ever want to erase it.

It has now become a part of my soul!

I called Debbie. I was concerned about her, about the doc with whom we share a history, the doc who led the charge that night. If you are familiar with the Trauma Junkie anthology, you have heard mention the name of Dr. Marson Ma; this former resident was one of Ma's residents, and I see Dr. Ma in him and adore him. Knowing he led the charge that day, knowing Debbie was working alongside him, helped me to realize that the doc's calm demeanor and brilliant mind gave this nurse, I'm sure, the confidence she needed to plow through. Good leadership, good ER docs, help nurses and medics do their jobs expertly, because if the doc believes we can do it, we can do it.

The phone conversation with Debbie occurred in my car on the way to Baltimore. The roads ahead were calm, weather beautiful, greenery, and hillsides breathtaking, all in sharp contrast to what Debbie was telling me. I asked her how she got through it, and her strongest response was about her family, her farm, her animals, her solace gained in that private sanctuary where she could mentally, emotionally, and spiritually sort out what happened.

Something that bothers me still is that a popular medical drama TV show of the time aired an episode based upon the incident Nurse Debbie Bowerman experienced in Las Vegas. In the episode, one of the nurses is performing CPR on a patient; she jumps on the gurney and is fighting for the patient amid chaos, blood, and death. The lead ER doc tells the nurse to stop, that she cannot save that patient, that there are others she can save. The nurse looks bewildered, then moves along to the next patient.

Oddly enough, that was Debbie's experience. Debbie's story. Someone took it and broadcast that incident, which you read Deb reference above, and plastered it on TV. We teach in critical incident stress management (CISM) that you can share your story, not anyone else's.

To take a very private and painful moment without asking permission is not cool. Tell your own story, do not tell mine or anyone else's without permission. Debbie authorized using a part of her story in this book; she wrote it. Debbie shares her experience from the aftermath of the 2017 mass shooting in public speaking engagements and conferences. She is still talking it out.

Verbal processing has always been a key point in my teaching crisis management from the 1990s to today; don't bottle it up inside, talk it out. If you think your family cannot handle it, talk to a peer support person, talk to your pets, talk to your truck, talk to the fish in a stream, talk to the wind. You need to hear yourself say words that will lead to sorting out what happened. And if all else fails, talk to a professional, but by Gosh, do not let an incident over which you had no control, that you did not cause, take your peace.

This is another example of folks still talking it out is through social media. Popular groups on websites or social meeting places crop up daily, usually divided by profession. One group wants evidence you were in EMS before the turn of the century (2000; we're not THAT old!). They share old pictures and ID badges, discuss algorithms, drugs, and equipment no longer used. They talk about how we used to playfully initiate new medics (Sean, I am sorry about hosing you down through the screen from outside while you slept in your bunk). We share a positive bond, of a time and attitude, from before people were quite so politically correct.

Back then, we talked about people who should be doing something, anything, else. They had bad attitudes, were not proficient, did not keep up on the medicine or protocols, would not give appropriate care, or start an IV because it meant a prolonged radio report and dragging the drug box through the hospital. They wanted the uniform and the glory (there was no/is no glory). They had an idealized vision of the job, and reality smacked them in the face with a short paycheck, long hours, and exhaustion from lack of sleep and too many shifts.

Those folks make interesting posts on social media. They make fun of patients and have absolutely no empathy. Some attack others for being less than intelligent; the war between levels of licensure existed then and is still prevalent. A doctor/nurse/medic must be stupid because they did not know "X." We do not know if the practitioner did not have an understanding of the procedure noted, but the complaining medic widened the divide by publishing his story, and those of like mind joined in on a tirade against common enemies.

Some folks take great joy in posting the positive things, the good memories, the reasons we are a secret society of oft-retired medics. We laugh about our foibles, about the guy who put his head out the window and made siren noises on the way to a call. We post pictures of candies in a biohazard bag, and parties with skeletons wearing uniforms, and party foods distributed in bedpans, emesis basins, and specimen cups (all unused, I'm sure).

We complain about our backs broken from lifting the old Ferno stretcher and marvel at the medics rolling around with hydraulic lifts. We remember people stealing long backboards from ERs or cutting off MAST pants. Just knowing about MAST pants and Ferno stretchers qualifies you as a dinosaur.

Then, in roll the fresh faces and modern equipment of today's emergency responders.

One of my recent professional endeavors was in a psychiatric hospital, mostly in addiction medicine. My roles were intake, and as a midnight charge nurse. Some of the medics shuffled in like Eeyore, moaning, and eye-rolling at having to deal with another nurse, another psychiatric patient. Playing my retired-medic, been-there-done-that card made them stand a little straighter, talk to me a little more kindly, and then share something amusing from a recent call. The bond was there, even though we had never met.

In retrospect, if only I knew then what I know now. Maybe I would have made smarter career moves, gone through graduate and doctoral studies earlier, spun the hamster wheel a little faster. Or maybe I would have slowed down during the frenzied times, realizing that the most important things were my family, my children, my sanity, my health, my peace.

Looking back is something we all do eventually. Erik Erikson outlined eight stages, and I am nearing the stage of "integrity vs. despair," which sounds devastatingly negative and getting ready for pushing up daisies. In this stage, we look at what we have or have not accomplished, experiencing possibly fulfillment or at least acceptance. Hopefully this stage brings with it wisdom from a life well-lived. The alternative is despair over not living a life we can be proud about.

Erik Erikson's wife, Joan, added a ninth stage, bless her heart. She addresses life into the 80s and 90s, a place I never imagined going. That final stage brings with it adjustments, new demands, and difficulties that include an aging, failing-the-war-with-entropy body. Looking back, I would take much better care of my back and have not such great pride in always being The Girl Who Could Lift.

So look forward, look back, but most importantly, look at the present moment. Be mindful of the exact place you stand without judging it. Feel the breeze. Smell the cut grass. Wiggle your toes in your shoes. Smile at the memories, look forward to the future, whatever it holds, and put your time and energy into that you cherish most while you still have it (or them).

My darling children, grandsons, sister, and furry babies, you give me great joy. When I look back, when I look at now, I don't see academic degrees, job titles, accomplishments, or the faces of patients that do fade with time.

I see you.

Glossary

Ambulatory: Relating to the ability to walk; not confined to bed.

Angiocath/IV catheter: The nasty needle that goes through your skin depositing a polymer tube attached to a hub that medical professionals use to deliver IV (intravenous) medications and fluids. The needle retracts from the catheter delivery system after successful insertion into a vein, leaving the flexible catheter in place; the hard needle does not remain in the vein even though the sensitized vein may feel otherwise and some patients swear, "It is still in there."

Arrhythmia: An arrhythmia or cardiac dysrhythmia represents a malfunction in the rate or rhythm (electrical conduction system) of the heart. Paramedics, who do not require calipers (measurement devices) to recognize abnormal rhythms because they see them so often, also tend to have slang terms for arrhythmias. You may hear AMF rhythm (Adios Mother F—er), CTD rhythm (Circling the Drain), FTD (Fixin' to Die), or an "Oh, 5hit" moment (replace the 5 with an S). No disrespect intended; see Gallows Humor.

Bag-Valve Mask (BVM): A hand-held disposable device with a bag, tubing, mask, and oxygen reservoir attached, used to provide positive pressure ventilation for patients who cannot breathe or cannot breathe adequately without assistance; also known as an Ambu-bag.

BFE: Slang acronym representing "Bum F— Egypt" indicating a very long way away. "They sent me to BFE and I did not clock out until three hours past end of shift."

BS Calls: Ambulance calls that some folks view as not merited, as when people use ambulances as public transportation without intention to pay for those services. BS includes such complaints as belly button lint, hangnails, and anything older than six months.

BS: Blue Sky (painting a pretty picture) also known as Bull Excrement (the acronym does not work as well, but it means the same thing), or Bull S—.

Caliper: A hand held hinged instrument with two pointy legs allowing for precise measurement (for the little boxes on an EKG strip displaying cardiac rhythms). A less precise method of measuring is counting the boxes (look at an EKG strip, you will see them), and most medics and ER staff can correctly identify rhythms at a glance. It is a science and an art.

Carbon Nanotube: A complex hollow carbon extension on an electron microscope allowing greater sensitivity in 'feeling/seeing' incredibly small particles of study (Nanooze, 2005).

Carotid Endarterectomy: The fancy term for a procedure designed to unclog the pipes (arteries) in the neck that permit blood flow to the brain.

Clearing (C-) Spine: The process of physician evaluation that determines no likely spinal injuries in a patient; this process is necessary before patients may be released from the confines of uncomfortable stabilization devices such as the long backboard or cervical collar (C-Collar).

Copious: An abundance or profuse amount of something; in terms of bodily expressions, it means a whole heck of a lot.

Delusion: A false belief often contradicted by evidence, can present as a symptom of a psychiatric condition.

Diaphoresis: Skin saturated with sweat, usually in response to a medical stimulus.

DSM-IV-TR: The DSM-IV-TR is an American Psychiatric Association publication: Diagnostic and Statistical Manual of Mental Disorders, fourth edition (IV), text revision (TR) in 2000, the mental health reference for standardization and classification of mental disorders. This is the best we have, until DSM-V solves all our problems.

Emesis: The product of regurgitation, vomiting. Slang: puke, upchuck, Technicolor yawn, tossing cookies, digestion recap, losing one's lunch, and so on.

EMT: EMT Basic: The first level of Emergency Medical Technician (precedes EMT Specialist and EMT Paramedic; each level bears progressively increasing skills, training, responsibilities, and licensure).

EMTP: EMT Paramedic: The top tier of Emergency Medical Technician, adding Advanced Cardiac Life Support (ACLS; also required of emergency nurses and physicians), extremely advanced skills, protocols, and lifesaving techniques. Many EMTPs also have other advanced certifications, such as Advanced Trauma Life Support (ATLS), Critical Care (CCEMTP), etc.

EMTS/EMTI: EMT Specialist/ EMT Intermediate: The second tier of Emergency Medical Technician, adding specific skills and medication administration abilities and responsibilities. Alpha lists always mess this up, but the progression order is EMT, EMTS/I, EMTP; the nomenclature may vary by area, and some states and agencies do not recognize the intermediate or specialist level.

Folie à Deux: Two or more unusually close people sharing the same delusion and supporting each other's beliefs (like an EMS crew). The delusion often develops because of the relationship people bear, and the development of the delusion in the second (etc.) party adheres to the context of the first party's delusion (Sharon, Sharon, Elijah, Shteynman, & Wilkens, 2009). Many in uniform call it getting through an impossible day, or coping with things people should not see or do, also known as... *life in uniform*. See DSM-IV-TR Diagnostic Criteria for 297.3 Shared Psychotic Disorder or the ICD-10 Diagnostic Criteria for F.24 Induced Delusional Disorder (*Folie à Deux*). Or say the heck with it and think, "Shared lunacy."

Gallows Humor: The coping mechanism employed by folks in highly stressful and traumatic situations that allows them to do their jobs without going completely bonkers. We are not making fun of really gross and intense situations, or the people they involve, we are just trying to get through what no one should ever see or experience. Making a joke relieves tension and makes things less real. Some say when you stop laughing you cry; we are too tough to cry.

Hemoccult Card: The specially prepared collection device upon which the doctor (or nurse) places a small amount of feces (poo) used to test for the presence of often-microscopic blood.

Hemoccult Developer: The chemical reagent dropped onto a hemoccult card the doctor (or nurse) uses to detect microscopic blood in the patient's feces (poo) sample.

Hemostats: Clamps (also called forceps) with a self-locking mechanism used by surgeons nurses and medics to control bleeding, as an alternative tool for numerous and sundry applications (including clamping off IV tubing cut accidentally by ill-placed medic shears when patient clothing is cut off). Also used by the public for holding small handmade cigarettes usually containing marijuana known as a Roach Clip.

HIPAA: Not "HIPPA" as with hippo: the Health Insurance Portability and Privacy Act of 1996 (P.L.104 -191) "provides federal protections for personal health information held by covered entities and gives patients an array of rights with respect to that information" (U.S. Department of Health and Human Services [US HHS], n.d., para. 1).

I&D: The acronym stands for Incision and Drainage, which is a surgical procedure (like cutting into and draining an abscess) performed with the ultimate intent of promoting healing.

Intubation: Intubation is the process of inserting a breathing tube through the mouth into the lungs to provide oxygen when the patient is unable to breathe effectively for himself.

IVDA: Intravenous Drug Abuse: illicit drugs such as Heroin injected directly into veins through a hollow needle (and syringe) for maximum effect. With long-term regular use and abuse, veins may become scarred and inaccessible (including between the toes).

KED Board (Kendrick Extrication Device): A semi-rigid device used to brace for stabilization and immobilization, usually by EMS or other rescuers.

LEIN/NCIC: Acronyms used by police officers; Law Enforcement Information Network, which is a statewide computerized information system, and National Crime Information Center, providing national computerized criminal justice information.

Lifepak 10: Portable cardiac defibrillator/pacer; used in the field and in emergency rooms for external cardiac interventions. The Lifepak 10 is an older model; technology has progressed significantly, so references identify archaic companies or really old stories.

Lividity: The bluish discolorations found in the dependent parts of a human body wherever gravity has allowed blood to pool. Also known as *livor mortis*, lividity contributes information regarding time of death and whether a body was moved (for further information, watch CSI).

Medic Shears: Serrated scissors with plastic grips able to cut through almost anything, including seat belts, leather coats, and heavy jeans material. Medics may say they have specially designed scissors that cut on seams to allow an experienced tailor to re-stitch expensive clothing, especially leathers, along the seams; this is an urban legend.

MVC: Motor Vehicle Crash, formerly called MVA, Motor Vehicle Accident. The word accident seemed to remove fault, a judgment; "crash" is a more factually descriptive word.

Mythomania: Excessive, habitual, or pathological lying; the word is not in this book, but it sounded so interesting it had to find a home in this glossary. So sue me.

Necrotic: Necrosis indicates tissue death, usually secondary to disease or trauma, and smells really bad, somewhat like the dead animals one finds along the roadway.

Newbie: Slang term to describe someone new in the business, comparable to a "probie" or "rookie;" one who is still in his or her probationary period, often as a new hire.

OCPD: Obsessive Compulsive Personality Disorder is a recognized personality disorder representing the throngs of folks who want things just so, who strive for perfection and success. Do not confuse OCPD with OCD (Obsessive Compulsive Disorder), a more pathologic expression. Many folks in emergency services (and other occupations) consider their OCPD a gift that keeps them organized and functioning at an impossibly high level.

OMG: Oh My God: an acronym adopted from young folks who wish to bastardize the English language for the sake of brevity and ease of texting or IM-ing (Instant Messaging; see your local teenager for further explanation). Multiple slang variations exist to express surprise, upset, distress, alarm, and amazement.

Pathological: Usually indicative of or relating to some physical or psychological abnormalities or disease processes, also known as bad stuff.

Plato's Cave: An allegory (symbolic story or parable) that proposes that we cannot perceive reality, but only its "shadow" or projection. You sit inside a cave with a white surface in front of you, but reality is outside. You can only see the shadows projected on your wall.

Precepting: Teaching or educating, giving the benefit of practical experience and training to a student, often used to describe an experienced staff member closely monitoring and training a newbie. Preceptors in EMS or FF often bear the title of FTO, or Field Training Officer. In nursing, preceptors pack and crack a hefty whip promoting "see one, do one, teach one."

Pretend-icitis: Loosely translated, pretend-icitis indicates faking appendicitis or any number of diseases warranting medical attention, sympathy from family and friends, and the opportunity to demonstrate personal acting skills. Pretend-icitis, unrecognized by the DSM-IV-TR, has been widely recognized by Gallows Humorists as inflammation ("itis") of the imagination.

Prison Wallet: Slang term for place of concealment used by male prisoners, also known as rectal vault. Squirming or wriggling while reading this explanation is perfectly normal.

Purulent: A medical term relating to a collection of pus, usually from a draining wound, and is thick, whitish (yellow, green, or brown), and foul smelling. Contrary to what I have seen medical students document, if something contains "pus" it is not "pussy," it is purulent.

Q Word: The dreaded Q word in EMS and ER is "Quiet," which wreaks havoc upon those in the company of the person uttering the word. Some declare this urban legend, folklore, mythology, or superstition. The "Q" word relates to the "S" word, "slow" (as in "slow night").

Rigor Mortis: The stiffening of a body several hours after death, not to be confused with a living patient who stiffens up because he thinks it will make him look sick (see pretend-icitis).

Ring Forceps: Surgical instrument (specifics vary, some are 6-9ish inches long) with circular tips used for grasping stuff during a pelvic foreign body removal procedure. Also used to hold belly buttons for piercing, a more likely place the public will see the ring forceps used.

Ross Bennett: An awesome comedian for over 30 years who takes a sidelong glance at timely topics; I can relate.

Sequelae: Possible secondary results or aftereffects of disease, injury, conditions, or event exposures; usually indicating some level of abnormality.

Spit Hood (or Spit Sock): A mesh, disposable, see-through protective device that fits loosely over the head of a patient (or prisoner) preventing spit from penetrating the mesh and reaching police or care providers. God bless its inventor.

Third-rider: An additional person (EMT, firefighter, doctor, or nurse) who rides along with an experienced crew (ambulance) hoping to gain field experience and training. Treat the third rider well and tell him it is policy for riders to buy the crew lunch; he may believe you.

Three Hots and a Cot: Slang term referring to three meals a day and a clean, sheltered, warm place to sleep courtesy of your local Emergency Room. Your nurses live to serve you. They will happily supply warm meals, ice water, fresh linens, extra pillows, and complimentary hospital footies. Forget getting a back rub, and do not ask how to order your free fruit basket as compensation for waiting too long to see a doctor.

TSS/Toxic Shock Syndrome: An uncommon but serious infection caused by *Staphylococcus aureus* bacteria or by streptococcus bacteria, which is a true medical emergency. TSS is sometimes linked to the use (and infrequent changing of) tampons.

Va-Jay-Jay: Slang term for vagina, uttered by the character Dr. Miranda Bailey of the television show *Grey's Anatomy*. It is a euphemistic descriptive more socially acceptable than using proper terms, reflecting the vernacular of the day and societal bastardization of language.

Voodoo (or Vodun): Voodoo is the dominant religion of Haiti, also practiced in some regions of the United States, and may involve animal sacrifice (Corbett, 1988).

References

Corbett, B. (1988). *Haiti: Introduction to Voodoo.* Retrieved from http://www.webster.edu/~corbetre/haiti/voodoo/overview.htm

International Critical Incident Stress Foundation. (n.d.). *Advanced group crisis intervention.* Retrieved from https://icisf.org/index.php?option=com_content&view=article&id=142:advanced-group-crisis-intervention-&catid=10:course-descriptions&Itemid=60

Nanooze. (2005). *The world's most powerful microscope.* Retrieved from http://www.nanooze.org/english/articles/article5_powerfulmicroscope.html

Richardson, J. A., Gwatlney-Brant, S. M., & Villar, D. (2002, February). Zinc toxosis from penny ingestion in dogs. *Veterinary Medicine.* Retrieved from http://www.vetmedpub.com

Sharon, I., Sharon, R., Elijah, J., Shteynman, S., & Wilkens, J. P. (2009). Shared psychotic disorder. Retrieved from http://emedicine.medscape.com/article/293107-overview

U.S. Department of Health and Human Services. (n.d.). *Health information privacy; HIPAA administrative statute simplification and rules.* Retrieved from http://www.hhs.gov/ocr/privacy/hipaa/administrative/index.html

Younger, O., Oeth, R., Taylor, J., & Cook, C. (2005, September 30). *Mississippi Katrina DR response: MS 35-05A after action report* (After Action Report). Retrieved from CAP Group 22: http://group22.net/katrina/Katrina.AAR.pdf

About the Author

Where did you grow up?
Born in Detroit and raised in its suburbs, I have lived with and around the economically challenged population most of my life; there is a unique perception of the world when you grow up poor. Fortunately, Mama was an Italian-American, Dad a US Marine, so the influences of my family (famiglia) taught responsibility, patriotism, and pride. The Midwest contributed a sense of connectedness and belonging, and the combination of community, culture, and ethics planted the seed of desire to become a patient advocate and agent for social change.

Why you are uniquely qualified to write this book
I can tell these stories because I have lived them and know the difference between dramatic representations and real life. Like many, I grew up watching the EMS and ER shows on television that focused on the hero aspect, providing predictable outcomes, and an unrealistic percentage of happy endings. Although television and movie depictions are more factual these days, the truth about how the emergency worker feels remains mostly hidden. My slant is in telling another side of the story: what responders think and feel during calls, how they internalize tragedy, what happens after the call, and how our world turns upside down when the patient is someone we love.

Why did you write this book?
When I tell people what I do, they focus on the gory side of life, like those who cannot look away from the scene of a bad accident. What they do not realize until it happens to them is that trauma affects someone who is loved and cherished, and lives are forever changed. I want people to see the world for a moment through my eyes, to walk with me through the broken glass, to sit next to me and hold the hand of the injured or dying, to fight against death thinking that sometimes we just might have the

power to win those battles. And then I want them to see the complete lunacy of it all and laugh.

What do you think readers will get out of it?

I am hoping that readers will see emergency service workers in a new light and realize we are human, too. We have our own challenges, pains, and sorrows. We have had surgeries, major illnesses, broken bones, and our share of emotional scars. We have been in accidents, our backs are killing us from lifting, and our feet ache after shifts that last from 12 to 24 hours, often without a break. We also realize the importance of last words, how sometimes the sound of an "I love you" has to last a lifetime.

One misperception I hear in the ER is that "you don't understand what I'm going through." Perhaps not, but folks may be surprised. Some may appreciate knowing what we think about after the call is over as we strip off our uniforms and professionalism, scrub off the bacterial and emotional accumulations of the day, and settle into an easy chair at home.

What will you do next in your life?

Things have changed dramatically in the past year. I work from home, and speaking engagements have been through video. CISM moved into teleconferencing, which is beyond me, so training is on hold. Despite heightened precautions in 2020, COVID-19 found me and left its mark; I am a fortunate and blessed survivor. I am writing and editing for the Michigan Crisis Response Association (MCRA), and editing into American English microbiology studies from a group in Italy (through Giovanni di Bonaventura, Ph.D., Professore at Università degli Studi "G D'Annunzio" di Chieti - Pescara).

The future is uncertain. I put one foot in front of the other, live an attitude of gratitude, watch, and improvise. Maybe this is how one eases into retirement, and in retirement, I hope to write.

Index

A

abdominal pain, 6, 18, 97
alcoholism, 54
allicin, 40
ALS, 17, 99
ambulance
    abuse of, 9, 10–11
    disturbing church, 67
    sex in, 20
    small town, 16

B

bedpan, 4, 75
Benadryl, 80
BFE, 66, 77, 78, 131
blowflies, 24
BS Call, 103

C

CAP, 1, 118, 139
Captain Hersler, 30–34
cardiac arrest, 63, 74, 80
cardiomyopathy, 62
cardiopulmonary arrest, 16, 104
catheter, 106, 131
Cerebrovascular Accident. *See* stroke
Chlamydia, 6
cholecystectomy, 75
chronic stress, 54, 116
CISM, iv, viii, 86, 88, 110, 112–16, 117, 119, 120, 122
Civil Air Patrol. *See* CAP
congestive heart failure, 63
Coughlin, J., 86
Critical Incident Stress Management. *See* CISM

D

debriefing, 110, 111, 114, 115
depression, 51
Detroit, 1, 12, 39, 61, 95, 109, 141
dogs, 84
double vision, 2
drug overdose, 68

E

earthquake, iv
EKG, 3, 10, 68, 132
emesis, 22
endarterectomy, 63

F

family
    as patients, 59
Folie à Deux, 133
Fort Campbell, 118
Fort Polk, 118

G

garlic, 22, 40, 41, 40–42, 42
Grey's Anatomy, 19, 137

H

hearing impaired, 90–92
heart attack, 3–4
hemoccult, 78, 133
HIPAA, viii
Hoover Dam, 71
Hurricane Katrina, i, 86, 117–23, 121, 139

I

I&D, 134
intramuscular injection, 94
intravenous drug use, 5
IV, 1–2, 70, 74, 101

K

King, R., 38

M

Ma, Marson, 127
maggots, 22
magic x-ray, 99–100
Mayo Clinic, 9
mindfulness, 26
morphine, 102
mucus, 23

N

newbies, 12–15, 30, 68

O

obesity, 10
orthopod, 77, 78

P

paramilitary, vii, 35, 65, 109, 112, 117, 118, 119
penis, 20
Peter Pan Principle, 67
pregnancy, 6, 8, 18, 39
pregnancy test, 6, 8
pretend-icitis, 97, 136
Prison Wallet, 19, 136
psychiatric patients, 50–53
psychiatric transport, 30–34
PTSD, 26, 27, 55, 118, 121

R

residents, 37–38
resilience, 25, 88, 107

S

scrotum, 17
seizure, 4
short coats, 38
sounding, 20
spit hoods, 44
stabbing victim, 80
STD, 3, 6
steroids, 77
stool sample, 7
storytelling, 113
stroke, 69
suicidal ideations, 47–48, 50–53

T

three hots and a cot, 99
Tompos, Bob, 30–34
tPA, 69

U

urination, 4, 8, 36
USAF, 112

V

vagina, 19, 41, 42, 137

W

warts, 36

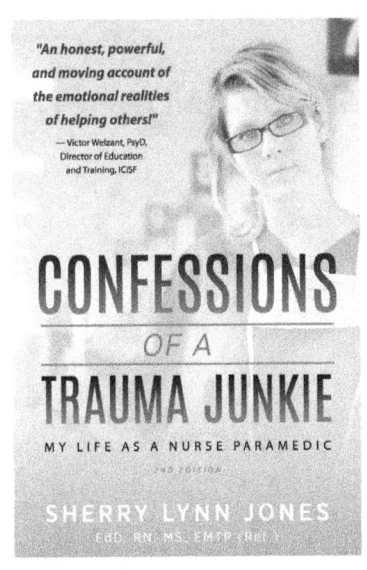

Ride in the back of the ambulance with Sherry Lynn Jones

Share the innermost feelings of emergency services workers as they encounter trauma, tragedy, redemption, and even a little humor. Sherry Lynn Jones has been an Emergency Medical Technician, Emergency Room Nurse, prison healthcare practitioner, and an on-scene critical incident debriefer. Most people who have observed or experienced physical, mental or emotional crisis have single perspectives. This book allows readers to stand on both sides of the gurney; it details a progression from innocence to enlightened caregiver to burnout, glimpsing into each stage personally and professionally.

"Corrections" is the third realm of emergency care behind layers of concrete and barbed wire. Join in the dangers, challenges, and truth-is-stranger-than-fiction humor of this updated and revised second edition of *Confessions of a Trauma Junkie*. In addition to stories from the streets and ERs, medics, nurses, and corrections officers share perceptions and coping skills from the other side of prisons' cuffs and clanging metal doors.

"Sherry Lynn Jones shares experiences and unique personal insights of first responders. Told with poetry, sensitivity and a touch of humor at times, all are real, providing views into realities EMTs, Nurses, and other first responders encounter. Recommended reading for anyone working with trauma, crises, critical incidents in any profession."
-- George W. Doherty, MS, LPC, President Rocky Mountain Region Disaster Mental Health Institute

Learn more at www.SherryLynnJones.com

Audiobooks available at Audible.com and iTunes

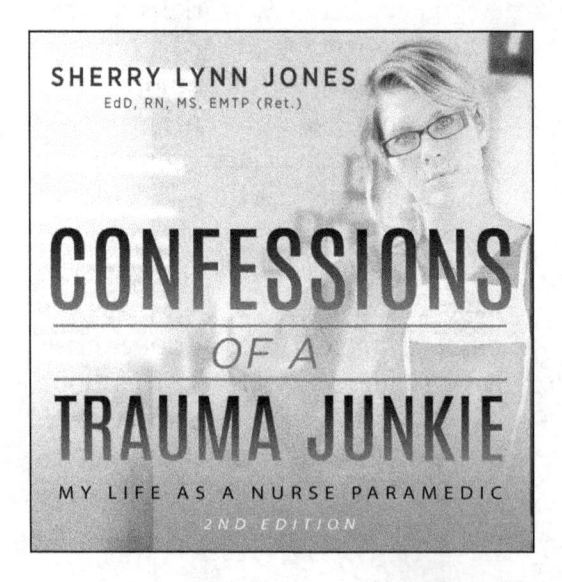

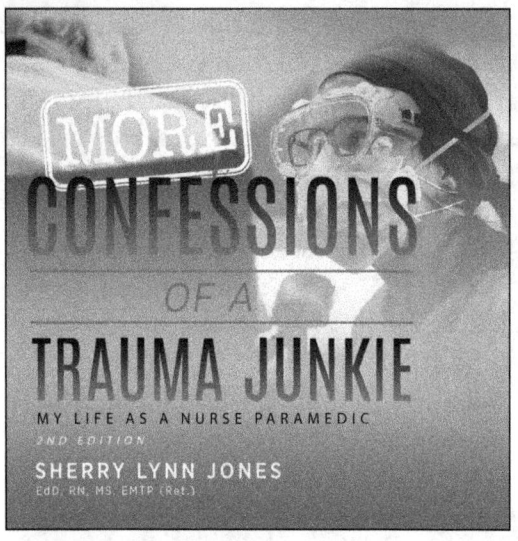

Recorded by Kris Bowen

Printed in the USA
CPSIA information can be obtained
at www.ICGtesting.com
CBHW071312140924
14521CB00039B/588